To My Parents

PREFACE

This book is designed to be read in a few sittings. It should acquaint, or reacquaint the practitioner with certain concepts regarding the care of psychiatric patients. The volume is designed to bridge the gap between research psychopharmacologic literature and anecdotal accounts of drug use as transmitted by teaching practitioners. Clinicians ultimately learn drug use through experience and the more mundane and practical issues of medication are not taught; it is the aim of this book to transmit some of those skills. I also wish to teach, concurrently, psychodynamic principles associated with drug administration.

This book was also prompted by the observation that there exists a dichotomy between those psychiatrists who practice psychoanalytically oriented treatment methods and those who use somatic therapies. Each perceives the other with skepticism and distortions. As in most things, conservatism lies at a midpoint. The basic thesis of the book is a coexistence of psychotherapy and psychopharmacology and I thus acknowledge the recent GAP Report on this subject (*cf.* p. 52).

This text represents my opinions. Minimal citations are included as basic references at the end of each chapter; the references are often review articles from which the reader can be steered to more information. Case examples form the pedagogic device for teaching. The reader will note that some psychopharmacologic principles are repeatedly made and that discussion of treatment moves from simple to complex issues within each of the first three chapters. A final fourth chapter deals with commonly asked questions and comments about drugs.

This book assumes a rudimentary knowledge of psychopharmacology. No dosages for drugs are given except in discussion of case examples. I have avoided detailed discussion of biochemical terms and omitted tables or charts in order to preserve the continuity of the text and facilitate its reading. Some logic of organization may be sacrificed for the sake of fluency; this is not a reference text but a volume to stimulate interest in a clinical subject.

Psychopharmacology is a science; its application to the treatment of mental disorders is an art. Knowledge of adverse reactions and compliance problems is necessary. Decisions about the withholding of medications are as important as the skill in titrating any drug dosage between inefficacy and toxicity. Symptomatic improvement is an end goal, but subtleties in patient functioning warrant the closest scrutiny by the clinician who elects to use psychopharmacologic agents in his practice. Such subtleties include cognitive functioning, self-esteem, and a capacity for growth and change. Drugs are thus viewed as adjunctive to the verbal therapies.

Help of the following people is acknowledged. Frank J. Ayd, Jr., M.D. graciously corrected many erroneous views I held about drugs and scrutinized early drafts of this book. Richard Sarles, M.D. and Leon Wurmser, M.D. gave their time to look at sections of the manuscript dealing, respectively, with drugs in childhood and drug abuse. Jose Arana, M.D. and Lino Covi, M.D., kindly helped me with concepts in the book regarding affective disorders. Joe Tupin, M.D. made helpful suggestions on manuscript organization. Russell R. Monroe, M.D. functioned both as reviewer of a portion of the text and, as Chairman of the Department, supported my sabbatical leave to undertake this writing; I remain grateful for this opportunity.

The book could not have been completed without the able secretarial assistance of Ruth Silvano, who patiently typed and retyped numerous drafts and gave me the benefit of her wisdom. Beth Dawson cheerfully aided by retrieving reference material and tracking down bibliography sources. Mr. T. Stevenson helped with the cover design.

This work was funded in part by a grant from the Foundation for Clinical Research in Psychiatry, Inc.

JOHN R. LION, M.D
Baltimore, 1978

CONTENTS

CHAPTER 1

Thought Disorders

This chapter will be concerned with patients who have thought disorders. Included among the group of illnesses are frank psychoses, paranoid conditions, and borderline states.

The drugs discussed in this chapter will be those referred to as antipsychotic agents. A variety of terms have been used in pharmacology to denote these drugs. Such terms include tranquilizers, neuroleptics, and psychotropics. The word "antipsychotic" will be used as specific for a generic illness.

A psychosis is a complex illness from the standpoint of pharmacologic control. The verbal manifestations of the thought disorder inherent in the psychosis are numerous. They include tangentiality, loosened associations, or incoherence. The behavioral components of psychosis are such parameters as psychomotor excitation and hostility, or retardation and mutism.

Disordered perception and cognition may appear as ideas of reference, grandiosity, or persecutory delusions and hallucinations. Generally, delusions and hallucinations which represent solidification of thought disorder processes are pharmacologically most resistant to change. Antipsychotic drugs affect first disorganized physical and verbal activity. Most of these activities are easily observed and hence useful for judgments of drug efficacy. More deeply ingrained and often insidious pathology such as systematized delusions require more detailed clinical observation and probing. In many instances, only the major behavioral responses are monitored in the treatment process and the patient is viewed as improved when he is quiescent. On closer scrutiny, cognitive and perceptual disorders persist, warranting continued pharmacologic therapy. The first case example illustrates many of these principles.

> A 16-year-old boy was hospitalized following a long illness marked by increasing defiance at his parents, decreasing interest in school, and the use of drugs. With time, he espoused mild persecutory delusional beliefs. He demonstrated psychomotor agitation with loosened associations and tangential thinking. He frequently giggled during the interview.
>
> Treatment was begun with trifluoperazine (Stelazine) 5 mg b.i.d. and increased to 80 mg within the first 6 weeks in the hospital. There was inadequate change in his condition and thiothixene (Navane) was substituted. This medication was titrated to 60 mg over a 2-week period. Upon receiving the second drug, the patient showed a greater response with decreased rambling speech and inappropriate affect. He responded to the hospital milieu and was discharged to outpatient psychotherapy.

This case illustrates the first psychotic illness of a young man whose premorbid history was that of social introversion. The psychosis was that of a moderately typical undifferentiated schizophrenic episode with some paranoid overtones. The episode may have had toxic origins or been exacerbated by drug use.

The question arose as to which medication to use for him and in which manner to use such a drug. In this instance, trifluoperazine was chosen as one of the more potent phenothiazines on a milligram for milligram basis. This class of compounds has less sedative effect; in fact, some clinicians claim this group of drugs to have stimulatory effects which have not been noted in careful clinical trials. One could have made a case for the use of a more sedating antipsychotic agent such as chlorpromazine (Thorazine) or thioridazine (Mellaril) since the patient did demonstrate some agitation and elation. Yet there was concern that he not be sedated for fear that the ensuing lethargy would make him more disturbed, not less. Adolescents cherish strength and virility. A sedative drug often causes more alarm, not less, as the patient feels drugged and apathetic. Fearing subjugation from others and experiencing anxiety, he intensifies his psychotic attempts to gain mastery over a loss of control. Viewed dynamically, some psychoses represent defenses against the breaking through of unconscious and unacceptable strivings for passivity within individuals who place a premium on masculinity and strength. While such speculations are not amenable to validation in early psychotherapy, they form a rationale for not rendering the patient inert and helpless through sedation. Had the patient been extremely agitated to the point of requiring a seclusion room, a sedating phenothiazine such as chlorpromazine or thioridazine might have been considered. No one class of antipsychotic compounds holds any advantage in the treatment of various types of psychoses (25). Chiefly, the sedative properties of the drug warrant consideration, if one excludes side-effects and toxic reactions which vary among the different classes of drugs. The clinician should recall, then, that antipsychotic drugs can roughly be divided into sedating and non-sedating groups. Most of the antipsychotic drugs developed early in psychiatry are sedating; newer agents are generally less sedating and more potent. Greater potency means that fewer milligrams are required to gain the same antipsychotic effect.

Trifluoperizine was prescribed for the patient in two divided dosages during the 1st week and then in one consolidated dose at night. There is a pharmacologic principle illustrated by this dose scheduling. It is now well recognized that the biologic half-lives of most drugs in psychiatry, with the exception of some antianxiety agents and lithium, are quite long (18). Antipsychotic drugs are stored in fat depots in the body and slowly released; after chronic dosing, metabolites can be detected for months in the urine. This fact forms the operating premise for infrequent daily dosing (16). Unless the patient is severely agitated and requires parenteral medication, the use of a t.i.d. or q.i.d. regimen is unwarranted when one is treating a psychotic patient with oral medication. Twice daily dosages facilitate adequate blood levels; after a few days or a week on such a regimen, the patient can be given the total dose before bedtime to facilitate sleep by capitalizing on what sedative properties the drug does have. Also, during sleep, neurologic reactions are less likely to occur. However, much has been touted about nocturnal dosing and there are some patients who are rendered so lethargic in the morning that divided doses are necessary.

Medication was given in liquid form. Several factors enter into the use of liquid concentrates as opposed to capsules and tablets. It should be realized that compliance rates both in and out of hospitals are notoriously poor, particularly if little attention is paid to the process due to large caseloads of patients and constraints of time. If the patient is mistrustful or frankly paranoid, pills may be taken unfaithfully. Some studies have shown that 50% of patients on a ward do not take their medication reliably (9). Patients who are given pills will secrete them in the pouch of the mouth and then discard them, save them up, trade them, or sell them. Liquid medication can also be "cheeked," and the patient can push cotton into the recesses of his mouth and tilt his head so that the medication becomes absorbed by the cotton which he can later discard. Regardless of the route of administration, patients should be watched to see whether or not they swallow the medication and a rinse of water or juice may ensure this with liquid drugs. Some medications are quite unpalatable in a liquid concentrate form and require supplemental juice. Alternately, there are some patients who require a medicinally flavored drug lest they feel they are being given nothing of value or a placebo. While certain antipsychotic medications such as haloperidol (Haldol) can be manufactured odorless and taste-less, their use in a surreptitious and secretive manner is to be avoided.

The disguising of medication carries a covert message of mistrust and reflects the ambivalence of the physician who prescribes or the nurse who dispenses the drug and prefers to avoid a confrontation with the patient. It is more direct and honest to inform patients why they are being given medication in a particular vehicle. It is also useful to have a dialogue with patients about the possibility that they may not like to take their medication because of feared adverse reactions or because they mistrust the medical staff. This often opens the door for meaningful discussion about the properties of drugs as well as issues of trust on the part of the therapist as well as the patient. Openness is always the preferred manner of handling drug administration.

Pills and tablets are more easily handled by patients who may be taught the responsibility of asking for them at appropriate times during the day. This is especially necessary for psychotic patients whom one is trying to resocialize by urging them to assume a more assertive and autonomous stance. Training the patient to ask for his medication is therapeutic; the passivity inherent in "medication time" where drugs are automatically handed out to all patients is regressive. Since pills must eventually be taken upon discharge, it behooves the clinician to induct his patient into the complexities of pill taking even though at some time during the patient's hospital stay he may well be on oral concentrate medication. Thus, in general, oral concentrates should be considered strongly in the early phases of acute psychotic management while pills and capsules should be used as a prelude to discharge. When compliance seems quite hazardous, long acting depot prepara-tions of the drug should be considered. This will be discussed in a subsequent section.

In the above case, trifluoperazine was titrated to a level of 80 mg with only limited effect on the patient. Disruptive behavior had abated, but continued evidence of a psychosis was manifested by inappropriate giggling and rambling speech patterns. The level of 80 mg was chosen as an end point in the decision to switch to another drug. The reasons for change were subjective and based upon a threshold fixed in the clinician's mind with regard to when a drug should or should not be working. Threshold decisions involve a time parameter and knowledge of what is considered a maximum dose to ascertain efficacy. *The Physicians' Desk Reference* (34) usually gives a conservative upper figure for "maximum" dosages. While this figure should not be taken as gospel for the maximum amount a patient needs or tolerates, it does give one a rough estimate of what dose should prove efficacious after a reasonable period of time. For trifluoperazine, 40 mg is a *Physicians' Desk Reference* recommended "maximum." This can be interpreted to mean that at that dose range some effect should be seen on the psychomotor manifestations of the psychosis within several days, and upon the delusions within several weeks. In the above case 40 mg was reached by the end of the 4th week without the desired change in the patient's status. Since there was no toxicity, the dose was escalated further. In the absence of efficacy after a total of 6 weeks, the drug was abandoned. Thereafter another class of antipsychotic agent, thiothixene, was chosen on a purely empirical basis.

Time and dose decisions are flexible. The trifluoperazine dosage could have been stopped at 40 or 60 mg, but no toxicity was observed. Thus, the drug increase was continued. Had toxicity appeared with increasing dosage, transfer to a new drug could have been effected earlier. The same holds true for time; *i.e.*, the clinician could have been more aggressive and reached 60 mg in 3 weeks instead of 4 or terminated the trifluoperazine after 1 month rather than 6 weeks. This may be the main criticism of management, for it appeared retrospectively that therapeutic attempts could have been more vigorous.

Time is an important variable. It has been shown that drug effects take time and there is a drug "lag" which may in part be based upon the slow buildup of the pharmacologic product in body tissues. Once drug effect occurs, the results are not linear but appear more logarithmic. A maximum effect occurs by at least the 3rd or 4th week of administration. Thereafter, one sees only small increments of change on any one effective dose. Figure 1 diagrams these observations. The

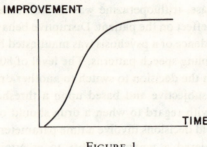

FIGURE 1.

graph reflects overall improvement; behavioral improvement occurs first.

The parameters followed for this patient reflect the need on the clinician's part to ascertain improvement through a variety of observations. First, one usually sees changes in sociability as drug effect takes place. The patient becomes less argumentative or belligerent, interacts more easily with others, and can sit still for ward meetings and other social activities. He may also begin to display a reduction in certain thought disorder symptoms of loosened associations, tangentiality, and inappropriate affect. Socialization is an early sign of drug response and nurses are usually the first to comment on the fact that the patient is "interacting more" with others. However, clinicians are often dismayed to see that this improved interaction is accompanied by no change in delusional content or the existence of hallucinations. Indeed, the delusions may persist quietly "underground" to the extent that the patient will not admit to them spontaneously unless asked. Thus, in many instances, improvement is deceptive. While the patient may deal readily with a variety of intellectural and social stimuli as a function of improvement from his thought disorder, a part of the psychosis remains untouched and may be visible only through more refined psychological testing or close clinical scrutiny. Unfortunately, detailed interviews are often sacrificed for the sake of time. It is at this point that the patient may be released from the hospital only to relapse from an imperfect remission.

On 40 mg of thiothixene, the above patient's thinking appeared more coherent. He attended group therapy sessions, making productive comments and even disarmingly perceptive observations about other patients. Incidentally, this should not necessarily be interpreted as improvement since psychotic patients are able to decipher primary process comments of other psychotic patients when they are sick. Nonetheless, the nursing staff informed the therapist that the patient was "better," and the therapist accordingly began to spend more time with him in individual psychotherapeutic sessions. It was there that he discovered that the patient showed residual psychotic processes. That is, the behavioral manifestations of the thought disorder had abated while the delusional-like material remained as yet unchanged by medication or the milieu. The patient related that he still felt others were "spying on me." Had this patient had hallucinations, he might have eventually confided to the therapist the fact that these also were intermittently present. Yet, such an expectation is possible only if one asks. Too often, there is a silent conspiracy to avoid inquiry about disturbing psychological issues. There exists a fantasy that queries about hallucinations will confirm the patient's anxiety about his "craziness," an anxiety he usually already has. This fantasy is similar to that involving questions about suicide and represents the idea that questions as to intent will plant the concept in the patient's mind and worsen the situation.

Having ascertained the patient's continued illness, the therapist increased his dose even higher to a total of 60 mg at which time the suspiciousness could no longer be elicited. Drugs should be continued despite a plateau of symptom amelioration to the point of further improvement, inefficacy, or toxicity. Toxicity includes the development of neurologic reactions, although these usually occur in the first few weeks of treatment. Other toxicities are sedation or confusion which can paradoxically worsen the clinical picture. Figure 2 shows the general curve picturing the relationship between improvement and

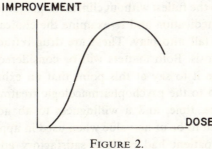

FIGURE 2.

drug dose. At some point, improvement can deteriorate due to adverse reactions, including depression or an organic brain syndrome from excessive medication.

When a different medication was chosen for this patient, the clinician gradually withdrew the trifluoperazine over the course of several days. Despite the long biologic half-lives of drugs in the body, abrupt withdrawal can lead to flu-like symptoms characterized by mild nausea and gastrointestinal upset. These symptoms may be reflective of the abrupt termination of an atropine-like effect of the antipsychotic agents which results in a rebound phenomenon; this reaction appears to be more pronounced if the antipsychotic agent is accompanied by an antiparkinsonian agent with cumulative anticholinergic properties. In any event, tapering is desirable for patient comfort. Antipsychotic agents should be withdrawn first as their effects and toxicities outlast the therapeutic effects of antiparkinsonian agents.

Multiple antipsychotic agents are generally to be avoided in the treatment of psychiatric disorders (26). All too frequently, the absence of efficacy of one drug makes the clinician decide to try another on top of the first with the rationale that there is a qualitative difference stemming from the addition. While the cumulative antipsychotic drug dose may be of value, such combinations may lead to cumulative toxicities and it is most difficult to determine which drug produced which effect, either positive or negative. The basic rationale of treating psychotic patients is to try one drug after another in an orderly and systematic fashion, titrating each drug to a maximum dose before viewing the drug as ineffective. Once so viewed, the drug should be discontinued and another tried. Of those psychotic patients who respond to medication, most will respond to the first two classes of drugs used. After a third and possible fourth class of antipsychotic drug has been exploited to the fullest without clinical improvement, the clinician should stop all medication and re-examine the clinical situation. Two possibilites then fall into play. These are drug refractoriness and an inaccurate diagnosis. Both matters will be considered in further case examples. Suffice it to say at this point that an exhaustive and systematic approach to the psychopharmacologic treatment of psychosis requires diligence, time, and a willingness to abandon those drugs which have shown to be of no value when used in appropriate dosage.

In time, this patient had made a satisfactory adjustment to the hospital and showed relatively normal thought processes. Some of his behavior was impulsive and erratic but consistent with his state as an adolescent. Whenever possible, the clinician must try to assess the premorbid state as the relative norm to which the patient should be returned. This assessment is often difficult. The family needs to be consulted for a description of how the patient has been behaving in the past. Some accounts of past history must be viewed cautiously for families often have a surprising tolerance for the deviance of a member and view him retrospectively as "always having been that way." Other families can give a more coherent account of decompensation.

The first case illustrated the utility of antipsychotic agents in the treatment of a patient with symptoms reflective of psychologic and physiologic activation—agitation, belligerence, excitation, and aggression. Outside of sedative drugs no one antipsychotic agent is inherently better for the treatment of these target symptoms than any other, despite claims seen in advertisements. Indeed, the impression that one antipsychotic drug may be useful for assaultiveness, while another is good for psychomotor retardation or autism has led to polypharmacy; the clinician adds a combination of drugs, each of which supposedly affects one target symptom in the overall picture. No research data support such an approach. Antipsychotic drugs suppress symptoms which lie on a continuum of pathology ranging from abnormal excitation to abnormal social retardation. The next case illustrates this aspect of use.

> A 23-year-old woman was admitted to the hospital following several days of progressively withdrawn social behavior. The husband would return at the end of the day to find the wife sleeping. The house had not been cleaned, nor had the children been adequately cared for. The patient was disheveled. On approaching her, she appeared suspicious and fearful. She occasionally spoke in answer to hallucinations, demonstrating ideas of reference, clang associations, and echolalia. She was often mute and remained by herself.
>
> It was felt that the patient demonstrated a psychosis with mixed paranoid and catatonic features. She was placed on trifluoperazine medication. Within a week, she became less seclusive and began to talk with other patients. Her fearfulness decreased and disordered speech abated. She ultimately made a recovery.

This case shows the utility of antipsychotic agents in "activating" or resocializing the patient. The features of drugs which decrease the abnormal excitation and stimulate retardation have led to the view of antipsychotic agents as "normalizers;" an analogy can be made to antipyretic agents which lower the temperature in febrile patients but not in normal people and to antidepressants which restore a normal mood in despondent patients but effect no mood changes in normal individuals. The concept of antipsychotic drugs as normalizers is useful in viewing them as being helpful in the treatment of psychotic states marked by apathy, autism, and psychomotor retardation. It is not difficult to understand the concept of normalization if one recalls that psychoses can manifest themselves in a variety of behaviors, each one in response to the altered perceptions and distortions inherent in the thought disorder of a particular patient (30). Which dynamics and defenses lead the patient to become angry, excited, or paranoid, and which lead to a posture of fearful apathy are unique to each individual. The antipsychotic drug exerts its effect on the cognitive and perceptual aspect of the psychosis with some concomitant reduction in any behavior reflective of that disorder. If the behavior is that of social withdrawal, this will be reduced so that the patient interacts more with others.

Some workers have commented on the psychodynamics of drug use and conceptualized certain drugs to free suppressed ego functions and repress disturbed id functions (33). For example, certain psychotic medications may suppress unacceptable drives such as anger in regressed and socially withdrawn patients who psychotically defend against the expression of rage by becoming catatonic. This formulation also explains the normalizing effect of antipsychotic drugs.

Once the acute phase of psychosis is under control, considerations must be given to the more chronic process. In terms of drug use, this is often labeled as the maintenance phase. The following case example illustrates problems arising during this phase.

> A 23-year-old man had been hospitalized with a diagnosis of schizophrenia. He was maintained on trifluoperazine 10 mg h.s. while being followed in an outpatient drug clinic. Upon a reduction in his dose to 5 mg, he became overtly psychotic with persecutory delusions and hallucinations. There was a positive alliance with the clinician in the clinic, and the patient complied with a return of medication to previous levels. Thereupon, his relapse was aborted and he was able to continue working.

Maintenance therapy is a topic receiving much attention in the literature. Studies have shown that 60 to 75% of schizophrenic patients relapse on placebo while only 25 to 30% relapse on antipsychotic medication (14). Thus, there is evidence to support the concept that retention on medication has prophylactic value. However, each case must be individualized. Opinions about maintenance medications have run the range of beliefs that patients with a psychosis warrant indefinite maintenance drugs to the idea that all patients deserve a drug-free trial. As in most things relating to patient care, an answer lies at the midpoint. A diagnosis of schizophrenia does not mandate years of antipsychotic drugs. There is a wide difference between drug requirements of a patient with one circumscribed "reactive" psychotic episode and the more chronically ill schizophrenic who has had numerous hospitalizations. Time, also, plays a role. Obviously, the more acute the psychosis and the more rapid its remission, the less one is likely to view the process as requiring long-term pharmacotherapy (19). It is conservative to take the view that an acute break in adolescence followed by a prompt remission warrants consideration of treatment without maintenance or with minimal maintenance interspersed with drug holidays.

In the above case the patient was placed on maintenance of trifluoperazine medication which was, over the course of several months, tapered. Upon the reduction in dose to a level of several milligrams he again became acutely psychotic. This relapse demonstrated his need for maintenance antipsychotic medication. There was a hazard that in the setting of a clinic he might be kept on maintenance medication indefinitely, since anyone scrutinizing his chart might become fearful of the consequences of dose reduction. This is a special hazard of drug clinics where medications and dosages are routinely perpetuated. All patients in such settings should be staffed at least annually and the continued need for drugs ascertained. An outside consultant is useful.

Patients are often urged to call the physician "if they feel bad," a well meaning statement which is superfluous without some introduction. Many psychotic patients have limited awareness of their illness and its ramifications and possess no guideline for the intelligent monitoring of their disorder. Yet such patients can be educated into the hallmarks of decompensation and alerted to recognize increased suspiciousness, agitation, or the intrusion of unwanted thoughts as indicative of the need for consultation or psychopharmacologic adjustments. In the above instance no such instruction was given and the reduction in maintenance medication resulted in the patient's becoming flagrantly psychotic. The time interval between lowering of the medication and the emergence of his psychotic relapse was approximately

2 weeks during which time the patient did not call the physician about his symptoms. While relapses are not explosive, they occur without the clinician's cognizance unless the latter is in a particularly opportune place to observe them. Only if the therapist is seeing a patient regularly (*i.e.,* once a week), does he have access to subtleties in mental status changes as a result of decrements in dosage. It also must be kept in mind that relapse, should it occur, will show itself up to 6 months upon discontinuation of the drug since all antipsychotic drugs, when used over lengths of time, are retained in the body for many months upon termination. Therefore, should the clinician decide to stop the medication, he must continue the patient in treatment and watch closely since decompensation does not occur immediately upon cessation of the drug. This may be an impractical arrangement in teaching and training institutions where there is regular staff turnover.

It was evident that the above patient might require maintenance trifluoperazine for several years given the exquisite sensitivity to relapse. Such a burden of requiring regular medication for a long time is in itself material for psychotherapy. Issues of self-esteem, reliance upon medication, the possible chronicity of illness, and its effects upon children, work, marriage, and sexuality are matters which need to be discussed but are rarely brought up in drug clinic situations. Spouses are often reluctant to interfere with therapy or are frightened to ask questions about long-term effects. When possible, conjoint sessions are useful. Any patient on long-term medication deserves the dignity of a prolonged interview which affords him and his family the opportunity to ask lingering questions. All can be taught about the emergence of subtle toxicities.

On thorough examination of this patient during one clinic visit, he told the therapist that he continued to feel that people were hearing his thoughts and that he was suspicious of the world around him. Coupled with this thought broadcasting were some auditory hallucinations in which the patient heard his mother calling him as he took a shower. He elaborated somewhat on the sexual nature of both the delusions and the hallucinations and it was obvious that the maintenance medication, while affecting sociability, had not fully suppressed delusions and hallucinations. In fact, rather than considering withdrawing the medication from him, one might consider increasing it to the point of diminishing the strength of these delusions and hallucinations. While they did not particularly bother him, the existence of such psychopathology represented ongoing schizophrenic illness which made the patient prone to relapse. An increment of dosage from 10 mg h.s. to 15 or 20 mg h.s. might be warranted, together with regular clinical assessment.

Opportunities for reduction in maintenance dosages may be indicated by insight which may come about through psychotherapy. A patient who can deal with issues of self-esteem or understand the nature of his autistic defenses may tolerate a reduction in dosage and the accompanying anxiety which can arise in the presence of intimacy. The patient who has developed introspection and can deal with homosexual strivings rather than handle them in a paranoid and projective fashion may have some capacity to grapple with his own conflicts to the point where medication may be tapered. These are long-term ventures requiring extensive output on the part of patients and their clinicians.

The "giving" of medication has strong symbolic value and is in itself a subject of psychodynamic relevance. A variety of views are possible. The patient may feel that medications mean that the clinician is not interested in listening, but wishes to avoid dealing with unpleasant verbal material. For other patients not receiving much of the doctor's time, value can be attached to the receipt of drugs, and pills can become the currency of care. While decrements in dosage may signify improvement, reduction paradoxically implies withdrawal of care and possible discharge (24). It may not be easy to discontinue medication in certain patients without risk of relapse. Such responses must be dealt with in psychotherapy to avoid the patient's shopping for a drug elsewhere. Increments in dose requirements are also problematic. While such increments may be alarming on one level, they may on another level be reassuring to a patient who craves continued nurturance. The point is that dose adjustments have their own psychological effects on patient behavior.

A general rule of thumb of maintenance medication is to continue the patient at one-third to one-fifth the amount he has required during the acute phase of his psychosis. The maintenance phase should be continued for 3 to 6 months after discharge and tapered slowly for a trial period. Periods of stress may require the reinstitution of medication. Such potential stress includes family discord, job difficulties, emotional losses, or physical illness. Prediction of decompensation is an important principle of maintenance care. The concept of prophylaxis can be taught to a patient and is conducive to a working alliance. The clinician might tell the patient that he appears to be going through a difficult period of time in his life and that it might be wise for him to be protected from excessive anxiety or depression during this time; the patient can be asked whether he would be willing to try a supplemental nocturnal dose of medication and relate whether this eases emotional functioning. Such a statement promotes collaboration by placing some responsibility for the medication on the patient and asking for his compliance. Dictatorial comments about "the need for more medication" or silent prescriptions handed the patient at the end of the session are demeaning.

The business of making patients a part of their drug management is time-consuming and not easily accomplished in large outpatient clinics or institutional settings. Indeed, the setting often shapes the model of interaction. In private individual psychotherapy for 50 minutes, fantasies about pills and drugs can be dealt with and explored. When a clinician is treating 20 patients on a ward, the model changes to one where drugs are simply dispensed without much discussion. One method of humanizing psychopharmacology in the latter setting is to have ward meetings to discuss only drugs and their effects and adverse reactions. Group meetings are also useful to deal with emotions evoked when one patient develops an adverse reaction. Fantasies and fears about potential short- and long-term toxicities or concerns about proper management by staff can arise (15). The matters should be aired openly, much as the disruptive behavior of a patient within a milieu would be discussed in group therapy. Tensions on a ward affect drug compliance and drug consumption (38).

A variety of clinicians have advocated depot preparations of antipsychotic drugs to assure compliance. This matter will be discussed later. Irrespective of route of administration, maintenance medication strategies must foster self-esteem. The goal of therapy should be to teach the patient to live with, titrate, and become knowledgeable about the need for medication. Many patients fall into passive postures with maintenance medication, and clinicians allow this to occur. Patients should always be urged to express their views on drugs and to describe their beliefs about drug dose adjustment. The patient must become aware of his illness and its manifestations. He must learn, since his psychosis may require long-term therapy, that adjustments in medication can be conjointly made between himself and the physician. This sense of autonomy helps in family interaction also. Whenever a family member is the identified patient, he can be subjected to manipulation by others who see him as controllable "if he takes his medication." If the patient has experienced the dignity of self-expression about drug requirements, he can withstand the family's pressures on him better.

Maintenance pharmacology requires documentation. Notes should include the rationales for treatment, dosages, side-effects, toxicities, and psychological changes. Regrettably, many psychiatrists are not good note takers and often rationalize this by stating that material told them by patients is confidential and should not be entered into any record. Psychopharmacologic treatment requires particular documentation not only for the sake of good practice but also for protection against possible malpractice liabilities. With maintenance therapy, months elapse before the clinician becomes aware that the patient has been on medication for so long. Only with adequate regular review of notes can wise judgments be made about decrements in maintenance medication or the need for consultation to monitor certain toxicities which will be described later. Notes should not be limited to the statement that the patient is "doing well" but should carefully describe his psychological functioning, the limits of his thought disorders, his social interactions, reasons for not titrating the medication further or decreasing it, and the anticipated length of time the clinician feels medication is warranted (10). On the front of each chart it is wise to write down each medication to which the patient has had exposure. In psychiatry, many drugs are the rule rather than the exception and by the time a patient has been in one facility and seen several psychiatrists, he has received many medications including one in the emergency room, one upon admission, several during his hospital stay, and one or more during discharge. While knowledge of drug exposure gives no indication of the success of such an exposure, it at least alerts the clinician to a drug history and enables a more intelligent decision to be made regarding future drug choices.

The patient described in the most recent case example was placed on an antiparkinsonian agent from the inception of his psychiatric treatment because it was feared that the development of a neurologic reaction might jeopardize therapy. The debate as to whether or not to start a patient on an antiparkinsonian agent to begin with centers about the efficacy of prophylaxis (17). This is an issue in paranoid patients or those with whom the clinician has a poor alliance and does not wish to frighten should the neurologic reaction develop. Yet studies have shown that patients not receiving antiparkinsonian medication are no more apt to have neurologic reactions to antipsychotic drugs than those who do receive both, although the severity of the neurologic reaction may be lessened. Antiparkinsonian agents appear to be most effective when administered upon the emergence of a neurologic reaction. The reasons for this phenomenon are not known; antiparkinsonian drugs may possibly be regarded as "normalizers" in the sense that they exert their effect on deranged states only.

Antiparkinsonian drugs can lead to an atropine-like toxicity manifested by confusion or psychosis. They may produce anticholinergic effects of blurred vision, dry mouth, urinary retention, constipation, and the exacerbation of glaucoma. Hence they are not innocuous drugs. If prescribed at all, they should be withdrawn after 3 months of use. The logic of such withdrawal relates to the fact that neurologic reactions occur most frequently during the early administration of antipsychotic therapy. Also, antipsychotic drugs are usually being reduced after 3 months anyway so that the patient receives a lower dose and incurs a reduced risk of a neurologic reaction. Even if a patient is placed on antiparkinsonian agents only upon the emergence of neurologic reaction, the drug should be experimentally withdrawn within several months to ascertain its continued need.

When antiparkinsonian agents are used, they should be given in divided dosages as their half-lives are not nearly as long as those of antipsychotic drugs. Most conveniently, it is useful to give them twice a day together with the antipsychotic agent. Antiparkinsonian agents rarely require rigorous titration beyond a few milligrams and the vast majority of neurologic reactions can be eliminated with these drugs in doses within manufacturer's recommended range. For the patient discussed above, 0.5 mg of benztropine mesylate (Cogentin) was used in the hospital and discontinued a month subsequent to discharge. All antiparkinsonian agents are equally effective. Antihistamines have been used to reduce neurologic reactions; these drugs are apt to produce sedation and are usually less desirable. As just mentioned, neurologic reactions are dose-related. Thus, reduction in antipsychotic drug dose may be as efficacious in reducing neurologic reactions as addition of antiparkinsonian agents.

One goal of reducing maintenance medication relates to the need to minimize the total milligram amount since long-term adverse effects appear to be dose-related. For some patients on low potency phenothiazines such as chlorpromazine, aggregate dosages over years may be in thousands of grams. Drug holidays or abstinence periods are used to reduce cumulative intake. Thus, medications are discontinued on weekends or given every other week with the rationale that blood levels will be sustained by drugs accumulated in body depots. With new higher potency drugs, fewer milligrams are given. However, drug holidays should still be attempted. Drug-free periods can be tried on weekends or vacations when compliance may ordinarily suffer due to disruption of routine.

Drug holidays may carry the covert message that "it really doesn't matter if the drug is taken." Hence patients who are feeling comparatively well will not see the need for continued medication at all. The clinician must address himself to this point and explain to the patient the rationale for an abstinence period. The basic aim of maintenance treatment is to use the smallest dose rendered over the longest length of time to control symptoms and prevent relapse. Toxicities resulting from long-term drug intake will be described later.

In both the acute and maintenance phase of treatment of psychoses, attention must be paid to the development of neurologic reactions. The propensity to evoke neurologic reactions is a common property of antipsychotic medications (21). The risk of neurologic reactions is related to potency of the drug. The older antipsychotic medications such as chlorpromazine or thioridazine induce fewer neurologic reactions while high potency drugs have a greater tendency to bring these about. Neurologic reactions are presumed to result from biochemical chances in striopallidal areas of the brain where these drugs localize. As such, they can be considered side-effects of the drugs.

Neurologic reactions have been called a variety of terms such as "extrapyramidal" or "parkinsonian." As antipsychotic medications produce cardiovascular, hepatic, and dermatologic reactions, "neurologic reaction" can be the generic term for the adverse effects involving discrete anatomical areas of the brain. Pharmacologic induced dysfunction in these areas generally produces changes in muscle tone and posture. Such changes range from a subtle rigidity and stiffness to the full-blown clinical picture resembling true parkinsonism.

The clinician must use some skills and have a sense of time fixed in his mind so that he can anticipate these adverse responses. The following case examples illustrate this principle.

> A 19-year-old man with a history of paranoid schizophrenia had been maintained on thiothixene medication up to 50 mg q.d. without antiparkinsonian medication. This medication had been discontinued within the past year, and the patient continued to function well in school. When fired from a summer job, he decompensated and showed increased agitation and paranoia. He agreed to take thiothixene, 20 mg h.s.
>
> Three days after beginning the drug, he called in alarm to state that his tongue was "falling in the back of my mouth—I have to stick it out." In addition, the patient stated that his eyes were "rolling around my head." While the patient's mother attributed these symptoms to his illness, they appeared to be dystonic reactions and disappeared within hours of his orally receiving 2 mg of benztropine mesylate.

This case shows the most dramatic and rapidly occurring neurologic reactions which are the dystonic ones, commonly manifested by tonic spasms of the muscles of the tongue, face, and neck; clonic spasms also occur and may be referred to as dyskinesias. These reactions occur mainly in young male patients. The onset of this reaction is within the first few days of treatment. Remission with antiparkinsonian medication usually occurs readily. Parenteral therapy with, say, 1 mg of benztropine mesylate given intramuscularly may result in dramatic amelioration.

Less rapidly occurring are the akathisias, manifested by diffuse motor restlessness of the entire body and extremities.

> A 35-year-old woman was admitted to the hospitale with a flagrant psychosis, necessitating parenteral medication during the 1st day. She developed a dystonic reaction on the 2nd day which responded to parenteral antiparkinsonian medication. Thereafter, she was placed on oral haloperidol (Haldol) 15 mg total daily dose; 1 mg daily dose of oral benztropine mesylate was also prescribed. The haloperidol was increased over the next 6 days to a total of 30 mg daily. By then, the patient's thought disorder had improved but she was observed to be pacing, complaining of an inability to sit still. She described an inner "jitteriness" which made her uncomfortable and stated that she had to constantly be in motion. Initially regarded as a transient worsening of her psychosis, the symptoms were eventually perceived as akathisic. They disappeared with an increase of the antiparkinsonian drug to 2 mg a day.

Akathisia is among the most distressing neurologic reactions induced by antipsychotic drugs. The above case illustrates these reactions which are notoriously insidious and vague, often closely simulating anxiety and agitation. Fears of impending doom or death may occur. Akathisias are most dysphoric to patients who make seemingly obtuse references to inner subjective states which are misperceived by clinicians and staff as part of the clinical picture of psychosis. It has been suggested that the akathisic reaction is one of the most important reasons that schizophrenic patients do not take medication (42). Hence, clinicians must monitor closely any occult or unusual symtomatology from patients receiving antipsychotic drugs. Antiparkinson agents may be administered on a trial basis to differentiate the neurologic reaction from symptoms of the primary illness.

After several weeks or months, one may see as a function of time and dose the picture of akinesia with muscle rigidity and immobility, rather than motor restlessness. Such reactions occur in middle-aged or older individuals. Akinesia may mimic depression because of psychomotor retardation. Response to antiparkinsonian drugs is variable, particularly if the clinical picture has consolidated over a lengthy period into the syndrome resembling parkinsonism with gait disturbance and tremor.

A final neurologic complication of long-term treatment are the tardive dyskinesias, reflected in hyperkinetic motions of the extremities, lingual, and facial muscles. The following example is illustrative.

> A 37-year-old man with a history of several hospitalizations for paranoid schizophrenia was maintained in an outpatient setting on 5 mg of haloperidol h.s. He appeared to be sensitive to this relatively small dose; attempts to reduce the dose to 2.5 mg had resulted in increased paranoid ideation and bizarre behavior. This dose had been given to him for 2^1/$_2$ years; he had received other antipsychotic drugs previously, but their nature was unknown.
>
> On one visit to the clinic, the mother complained that the patient was making strange movements of his mouth. The patient himself usually sat with his hands cupping his chin in a natural pose, so that the mouth movements were not easily visible. Upon removal of the hand, he displayed a puckering of his lips and sideways smacking-like motion of the jaw. He attributed this to new dentures. On inspection of his tongue, vermicular movements were noted.

The above case is illustrative of a tardive dyskinesia. The onset is early; most cases appear in elderly females who are at higher risk. The patient had been on comparatively little antipsychotic medication for a long period of time and was evidently sensitive to the drug. Yet, retrospectively, one might wonder whether the patient fully required the maintenance dose for such a long period or whether drug holidays could have been tried. One point to be made by the example is that tardive dyskinesias are in part idiosyncratic. While usually seen in older patients exposed to high doses of low potency antipsychotic agents, they can develop in younger patients with less drug exposure who somehow are biochemically predisposed to the complication (4). Thus, it behooves the clinician to aim for the lowest maintenance dose, to experiment and document drug reduction or withdrawal, and to monitor the possible emergence of the dyskinesia by inspecting the tongue for difficulties with sustained protrusion or fine rhythmical movement. Involuntary movements of the fingers or frequent eye blinking may also herald toxicity.

Interestingly, the above patient denied the dyskinesia, stating that it was part of his associated dental irritation. This is not unusual. Unlike dystonic reactions which are often painful and physically obvious, dyskinesias are subtle and appear insidiously. The patient often incorporates symptoms into his behavior, making such symptoms syntonic and refusing to view them as toxic in origin. Parents or other people are often the first to notice. The opposite is true of dystonic reactions where the patient himself is acutely aware of the reaction.

The above case was problematic. No definitive treatment exists for tardive dyskinesia. Antipsychotic drugs mask the symptoms and most tardive dyskinesias are discovered upon cessation of the drug or reduction in dose. Some may be reversible, particularly those seen in young patients (35). Early dyskinesia as manifested in lingual or digital movements may remit with time. "Breakthrough" dyskinesias appearing while the patient is on antipsychotic medication are often more ominous, usually being less reversible. Such conditions pose an ethical dilemma for the clinician. Continuation of pharmacologic treatment may keep a dyskinesia under temporary control yet possibly worsen the condition in the long run. Should drugs be reduced or withdrawn, psychotic relapse may ensue. There is no simple solution to this problem (8). A change to another high potency antipsychotic drug which may be less likely to induce tardive dyskinesia could be considered. Alternately, a depot preparation which offers even lower milligram dosages could also be another choice. In all instances, the decisions and risks must be shared with the patient and documented in the record.

Despite the fact that acute neurologic reactions can be reduced or rapidly abolished by dose manipulation or by the addition of antiparkinsonian drugs, patients understandably have an emotional response to an antipsychotic drug which produces such a bizarre effect and are often loathe to continue taking the medication. In the case of dystonic reactions, reassurance is necessary and the patient must be told that such reactions are not uncommon and can be controlled. It behooves the clinician to monitor the patient closely during the first days or weeks when he begins a patient on antipsychotic medication. In hospital settings, physicians are usually available and the etiology of the dystonic reaction can be elucidated. In outpatient settings, however, patients who are not educated may immediately rush to an emergency room where a misdiagnosis of catatonic schizophrenia, tetanus, or meningitis can be made. Traumatic diagnostic procedures may be performed. It is incumbent upon the physician to advise the patient and family of the possibility of the development of a neurologic reaction. In the case of reliable patients, some antiparkinsonian agent can be given in a small envelope to be used "for muscle stiffness" although the clinician might prefer that the patient contact him directly in order that he might rule out psychological variables. In all cases, prescriptions should be labeled and a card should be carried by the patient in his wallet identifying which drugs he is on since patients often leave their medications at home. This card should not simply be handed to the patient but should be discussed with him.

Akathisic and akinetic responses confuse the patient by virtue of producing motor restlessness or muscle stiffness which the patient does not clearly identify as a reaction to the drug. These drug-induced reactions may worsen the patient's condition. Education ahead of time is necessary.

Some clinicians feel that patients should be spared the worry of such long-term toxicities since they are already troubled sufficiently by their illness. Also, mention of toxicities may frighten such patients into noncompliance. Neither perception is fully accurate. Patient can be told of potential complications in a manner which allays anxiety; not every adverse reaction needs to be spelled out. For example, it is entirely premature to tell a patient about the risk of tardive dyskinesia at the inception of drug therapy since the duration of treatment is still unknown. After several months of continued drug use, the topic can be brought up.

The parenteral use of antipsychotic drugs is often necessary in acutely agitated states as illustrated by the following case example.

A 23-year-old female was brought to the emergency room because of bizarre and agitated behavior. She was talking loudly and defiantly at her relatives. She was alternately euphoric about some mystical experience and would then sob relentlessly. Her speech was disorganized and she demonstrated pecular posturing which apparently was in response to some religious convictions and voices. She paced back and forth and was hostile and negativistic.

Because of the acute agitation, a dose of 5 mg of haloperidol was given intramuscularly. One-half hour later she showed a diminution in her boisterousness and hyperactivity. However, posturing and delusional activity persisted and an additional 5 mg was given to her parenterally 30 minutes after the first dose. Subsequent to this injection, the patient appeared more cooperative and demonstrated no agitation or anger. She was admitted to the hospital and begun on oral haloperidol medication; the regimen was 10 mg t.i.d. On the evening of the next day, 24 hours after admission, she demonstrated a neurologic reaction with nucal rigidity. This dystonic reaction responded to 2 mg of benztropine mesylate given intramuscularly. Thereafter the oral dose was continued at 8 mg t.i.d together with antiparkinsonian medication until discharge.

The more widespread use of the high potency drugs has generally supplanted low potency agents for emergency room use. Parenteral chlorpromazine carries with it the hazard of hypotensive reactions and excessive sedation. Haloperidol is a potent antipsychotic agent which can be given to acutely agitated patients without risks of hypotension and sedation. Excessive sedation is undesirable for the same reasons mentioned earlier; that is, it may exacerbate a patient's fear of loss of control (5). While it is a mistake to overwhelm the patient with sequential injections of an antipsychotic drug until organic and toxic etiologies for the psychosis are ruled out, the patient must obviously be tractable in order for a history and physical to be carried out. Hence, the clinician is often quite justified in giving one calming dose with cognizance of the fact that an additional evaluation is necessary. Documentation to this effect should be placed in the chart.

Much has been written about the use of "chemical restraints" in preference to physical restraints. Most clinicians feel that the physical handling of the patient with sheets, cuffs, or other devices which would bind him to a stretcher are anachronistic and punitive. This assumption needs to be questioned. The humane use of physical restraints together with talking is an effective way of calming an agitated patient who may be violent (31). The availability of potent antipsychotic agents does not preclude the need for any medical facility to have on its staff professionals who are trained in the management of agitated patients and who can at times physically subjugate such patients when necessary. It is often dangerous to approach a very agitated patient with a syringe in hand.

Agitated patients who have received parenteral medication are often immediately transferred to wards and seclusion rooms while the antipsychotic medication takes effect. The employment of parenteral medication gives the physician an opportunity to do some therapeutic work with the patient during a more quiescent phase. Patients who are acutely agitated may reveal their anxieties when calmed by the drug. This gives the clinician a chance to ascertain the nature and existence of the delusion or hallucinations or to sharpen his diagnosis. Too often, the simple reduction in agitation and motor excitement is seen as the end point for parenteral medication while no attention is paid to the acquisition of anamnestic material during the patient's calmness. In some instances, the psychodynamics of the psychosis can be exposed during the phase of parenteral antipsychotic administration provided that the clinician spends time with the patient and has an interest in this process. Exploration of psychotic content should be done in a nonconfronting manner so as to not excite further the patient who is attempting to cope with alien thoughts and fears.

A psychosis, particularly an acute one, is a highly dystonic affair for most patients who retrospectively recall the terror and anxiety. The abolition of acute suffering of psychosis, together with the need to restore the milieu in an emergency room or ward setting are the main indications for parenteral drugs. Some clinicians have proposed that parenteral drugs may effect a more rapid resolution of the psychosis (3). There is no clear evidence for this claim. The rapid calming properties of parenteral medication do, however, induce cooperation in patients and enable them to establish rapport with staff and certain hallmarks of psychosis such as hallucinations and delusions may be sufficiently suppressed through the use of parenteral medication to facilitate a smooth transfer to a ward setting.

Parenteral medication is a dynamically important form of treatment

suitable for transfer to an inpatient setting. Any patient who is acutely psychotic to the point of requiring parenteral medication generally requires an observational period in a hospital for continued treatment. In rare instances, when beds are unavailable and finances dictate otherwise and there is a strong family network, patients can be discharged to home with continued oral supplemental medication and follow-up by an office visit the next day.

It is undesirable to titrate to the point that the patient becomes inert. Clinicians should be aware, however, of the fact that once pharmacologic control over a psychosis has been achieved, the patient may go to sleep. Such sleep is interruptable and does not have the drugged quality to it. The need for sleep probably represents sleep deprivation due to psychosis and is generally a healthy sign, indicative of some mental restoration.

Once maximum calmness and cooperation is reached and the end points of reduced motor excitation and agitation are observed, oral medication can be used. In the above case, oral medication was begun the evening of admission, 6 hours after the last injection. There is no specific time duration to wait for initiating oral medication since entry into the circulation will be delayed and time is required for attainment of subsequent blood levels. Various clinicians have advocated oral medication to be from 1½ to 3 times that required during the parenteral phase. Thus, the above patient received 10 mg by injection and 30 mg during her daily oral medication phase. The fact that higher amounts of oral medication are needed results from delays in absorption. Oral medication should be given in either a single nocturnal dose or divided doses but rarely needs to be given more than twice daily; in the above example a t.i.d. regimen was unnecessary.

Oral medication following parenteral administration is often referred to as the "oral maintenance phase." This is probably a misnomer. The medication requirements of the patient subsequent to the parenteral phase illustrates his needs during unresolved illness and are not representative of a maintenance drug level required for the period during remission. Indeed, during the switch over from parenteral to oral medication, the clinician may note that while the patient is calmer and more manageable, the delusions and hallucinations may persist and even become stronger and more solidified. In such instances, a flexible approach should be maintained with options to raise the oral medication to a more appropriately therapeutic level.

Attention will now be directed toward the development of neurologic reactions. While neurologic reactions can occur at any time during the administration of an antipsychotic agent, they are generally less common during the use of parenteral drugs than during oral treatment. The reasons for this are unknown but may relate to parenterally induced higher blood levels with a concomitantly higher anticholinergic effect; the drug may act as its own "built-in" antiparkinsonian agent (41). Neurologic reactions occur 12 to 48 hours after parenteral administration and often become visible on the ward when oral medication is being used, as was the case in the above illustration. Dystonic reactions are the most common. In rarer instances, akathisia may be seen after the parenteral phase. Because the development of neurologic reactions is delayed, attention is often withdrawn from the patient during the time he is quiet and being integrated into the ward. It is important for the clinician to alert his staff and to have appropriate medication orders and resources available to administer antiparkinsonian agents should reactions occur. Antiparkinsonian drugs can be used parenterally to control acute dystonic or akathisic reactions as they emerge.

There is no evidence that parenteral antipsychotic medication makes neurologic reactions more severe; the fact that such reactions occur when they are least expected after the acute phase often makes them appear more dramatic only (6). Once again, antiparkinsonian agents may be given prophylactically to certain paranoid patients, but it should be recalled that they have limited efficacy. Antiparkinsonian agents have their own toxicities which can cloud the clinical picture.

Older patients may react adversely to parenteral antipsychotic agents and small dosages should be used, such as 1 or 2 mg of haloperidol. The drugs of the benzodiazepine class such as chlordiazepoxide (Librium) may be safer as they are eliminated from the body more quickly, although they are absorbed erratically from intramuscular injection sites.

Not all patients are candidates for medication, despite the fact that they are ill. The following case illustrates this problem.

> A 22-year-old man demonstrated bizarre behavior following rejection by a girlfriend. He felt compelled to set fires to trash on the street, believing he had talked with emperors, kings, and other important people

in the world and was sent to America to clean up pollution. He was hospitalized for a few days and received a few doses of thioridazine, then transferred to another hospital where he promptly reconstituted without evidence of delusions or hallucinations. He engaged in outpatient therapy twice weekly, and demonstrated mild paranoia. He initially was seclusive and remained at home all day, watching television and reading. After many months of treatment, he became more sociable and left his home to take work in another city. The therapeutic alliance was strong in the face of chronic mistrustfulness and suspicion that could be easily elicited in therapy sessions.

This case shows the difficulties confronting clinicians who treat paranoid or borderline individuals on an outpatient basis. In many instances, medication cannot and probably should not be given because the patient refuses it or views it as a focus for a power struggle between himself and the therapist. Paranoid patients preoccupied with masculinity often do not like the passivity inherent in drug taking and, as mentioned earlier, respond to lethargy or any of the subtle neurologic side-effects induced by antipsychotic agents with alarm and hypervigilance and intensify their paranoid stance (39). The clinician was convinced in the above case that the administration of an antipsychotic agent for the purpose of reducing the suspiciousness of a residual psychosis might in fact exacerbate the patient's illness and erode a therapeutic alliance which was initially delicate.

Many paranoid patients use projective defenses to convert inner anxieties and feelings of worthlessness into accusatory threats. No drug treats the lack of trust and inner emptiness even though there are medications which are effective for the treatment of the pervasive anxiety of these individuals. A point exists, then, for the use of antianxiety agents such as the benzodiazepines to treat certain paranoid patients. These drugs have far fewer side-effects and when given in conservative amounts, do reduce anxiety. They have potential to cause mild sedation, but the sedation is qualitatively less profound than that induced by antipsychotic drugs and often more acceptable. Subtle neurologic reactions are absent.If the above patient was worse than he actually was, diazepam (Valium) or chlordiazepoxide might have been a useful adjunct to psychotherapy. However, the therapist must make the entire issue of medication highly negotiable with the patient so that the latter has the feeling of some control over his therapy given the fragile nature of the alliance. Medication must never be thrust upon paranoid patients. Instead they should be asked whether or not they think medication might make them more comfortable. Questions regarding drugs are usually accompanied by negativism indicative of the concerns described above. The clinician must respond to such concerns directly and without evasion. The name, properties, and expected results of the drug should be outlined to the patient so that the latter sees this as an open therapeutic gesture. Some paranoid patients have a remarkable ability to learn about the side-effects of drugs and will look up the name of medications or gain access to pharmacology texts. If such a move is suspected, patients can be given a reference on psychopharmacology and on occasion even be shown the *Physician's Desk Reference* so that they can read about the drug. While the latter book contains a comprehensive list of toxicities and side-effects, the openness of the process often transcends any alarm attendant to viewing the contents and helps gain trust.

The clinician's posture with regard to the above patient was to await his return to society with the intrinsic belief that he had the ability to find a job. This idea, covertly conveyed to him by waiting and listening, was worth more than any medication. His regressive and autistic withdrawal at home was indeed alarming to the parents, but the patient himself was aware of his suspiciousness and fearfulness and could freely talk about it. Because this patient was articulate and the therapist eventually developed a good rapport on a twice weekly psychotherapeutic basis, the anxieties could be verbalized and certain distortions corrected. Delusions or hallucinations could never be elicited. Had they existed, small amounts of antipsychotic medication might have been warranted.

It has been pointed out that patients respond to medication in the same way that they react to other events in their life (23). Those who crave medication often have an insatiable need for nurturance while those who are disdainful and resent pills respond the same way toward authority figures in society. The above patient was an example of this. He saw pills the same way he say his parents and society at large and tended to be antagonistic, rebuffing attempts at kindness and nurturance in the service of toughness and independence. This toughness was a veneer; in time, it could be pointed out to him in treatment. Medication would have undercut a subtle belief his therapist displayed that the patient could make it on his own. The need to adhere to this belief is often prevalent among adolescents who are cherishing independence and masculine prowess at the same time they are struggling with the issue of dependency on their own parents. It is known that compliance among adolescents is poor not only with psychopharmacologic agents but with other drugs such as insulin or anticonvulsants. Counterphobic attitudes toward medication cause such patients to abandon them. Also, the social awkwardness of carrying pills becomes embarrassing. Finally, there is a need on their part to relinquish medications once they "feel better," a behavior not only limited to adolescents but to the general population at large. All these issues must be addressed in psychotherapy.

There are certain paranoid patients who demonstrate such marked overreactiveness and lability of affect and behavior in response to minor stresses that antipsychotic agents are warranted as drugs of choice. Generally, the tack would be to utilize small amounts of a non-sedating agent such as trifluoperazine. The patient can be started at a very low dose range and counselled to the fact that this particular medication may do nothing; in that event, the dose will be increased. This is wiser than starting with a larger dose and running the risk of inducing a side-effect which severely hampers therapy and the patient's tendency to comply with future drug regimens. Certain labile paranoid personalities will tolerate 2 mg of trifluoperazine given twice daily or 4 mg at night; prophylactic antiparkinsonian agents may be used if the daily dosage reaches 10 mg. It is wiser to prescribe antiparkinsonian agents since it is precisely this diagnostic group one wishes to avoid frightening.

The rationale for using antipsychotic agents is to reduce excitation and agitation which has a psychotic flavor to it while at the same time abolishing some anxiety. While it is often claimed that antipsychotic drugs have no antianxiety properties, this is not precisely true. The antipsychotic agents most certainly have a quiescent effect. However, they should not be used for anxiety which can be treated with less toxic agents; the issue is the risk of using an antipsychotic agent more than the academic argument of whether or not it produces an effica-cious reduction in the patient's anxiety. Along these lines, it must be recalled that paranoid personality traits and paranoid psychoses are on a continuum ranging from simple suspiciousness to complex delusions. As a paranoid condition worsens, perceptions of the environment and the cognitive responses to them are qualitatively altered and approach a true thought disorder. Thus, antipsychotic agents do have a place in the management of a paranoid individual when used before the development of a paranoid psychosis. Alternately, a point can be made for the safer treatment of paranoid anxiety with antianxiety agents. When to use antianxiety agents and when to use antipsychotic agents in small amounts must remain a matter of clinical judgment and is in part dictated by the patient's attitude and the degree of suspiciousness and distortion.

In the above case, the patient ultimately took a job. He was subjected to some criticism by his supervisor. He responded to such criticism with anxiety and anger which appeared to be of non-psychotic proportions. While no medication was prescribed during psychotherapy, his therapist could have conceptualized the anxiety as detrimental to his functioning in the sense that it might have increased his hypervigilance to psychotic proportions. Hence, an antianxiety agent could have been given to him; with increased hypervigilance and paranoia, an antipsychotic drug could have been chosen. Many paranoid patients can be made to see their suspiciousness. Paranoia is a relatively dysphoric condition often recognized by the patients as a need to always be watchful. Certain patients will be the first to admit that they "carry a chip on their shoulder" or are always "looking out for the other guy" or perceiving the world as unfriendly. The chronic level of their vigilance can never be relaxed and betrays certain insecurities. However, while most patients would wish for a reduction in their need to always watch out for the other guy, they will not take medication precisely because it makes them succumb to the very forces they fear. If medication is given at all, it may be left with them to titrate the dosage. The physician can prescribe guidelines but not insist upon a fixed regimen lest it make the patient feel trapped and helpless.

Physicians too often assume authoritarian attitudes. They are often uncomfortable with the negotiation of medications with patients and see such discussions as a threat to their professionalism (24). Yet for many patients, the opportunity to engage in dialogue with the physician about medication the latter wishes to prescribe may represent the first time that a patient has ever seen a positive outcome resulting from a difference of opinion—an outcome unaccompanied by physical altercation or the withdrawal of affection. An authoritarian stance or posture is counter-productive in the management of paranoid patients. It can be pointed out by the clinician that an optimal dose would be twice a day but that the patient is in control of his medication and "is in charge." More is accomplished by such an attitude than by the dogmatic recital of dire consequences.

As problematic for pharmacologic therapy are borderline patients. This is illustrated by the next example.

> A 24-year-old single girl was seen for consultation following the failure of 2 years of intensive psychoanalytic therapy to modify her behavior. The patient's difficulties were addictive traits and drug abuse, mood lability, and regressive psychological functioning. She had been unable to find stable employment and was prone to miss work, plagued by many hypochondriacal symptoms including nausea and vomiting for which no organic basis could be found. Often, she had many phobias, episodes of depersonalization, and periods of hallucinatory-like behavior. She made several suicide gestures when romantic relationships failed.
>
> Over the course of several years treatment, she had seen six psychiatrists and had been prescribed at one time or another four antipsychotic agents, three antianxiety agents, lithium, two types of hypnotics and two types of anticonvulsants. Despite the vast array of medications given her, there appeared to be consensual validation by all clinicians that she was a typical "borderline" girl.

This case is not atypical for so-called borderline. The terms "borderline," "latent" schizophrenic, "ambulatory" or "psudoneurotic" or "psychotic character" have been used interchangeably in clinical practice and the vast literature on this subject has lacked cohesive criteria for the diagnosis. Currently, DSM III formulations utilize the term "Borderline Personality Organization" (2). There have been few studies on the psychopharmacologic treatment of borderline conditions (29). One set of workers have chosen to view the particular symptom complex of emotional lability prevalent in these patients and treated them with lithium carbonate. Yet these patients are often unreliable and this makes lithium carbonate a hazard in therapeutic use; since lithium must be taken regularly and will be toxic if not taken appropriately, it is not the best pharmacologic agent to give patients who show emotional instability. In addition, lithium has little "quenching" action. Most medications produce some degree of sedation or relief from anxiety or tension and it is those drug properties which the borderline patient often craves.

Antipsychotic agents may also be seen as drugs of choice for these patients who are conceptualized as having many psychotic features. Unfortunately, borderline patients are often preoccupied with body image and bodily sensations so that antipsychotic agents are discarded because of their numerous pharmacologic side-effects and toxicities (39). Neurologic reactions of muscular rigidity or subtle akinesias or akathisias are intolerable for borderline patients who are prone to episodes of depersonalization. The reactions vastly accentuate the anxiety and worsen, rather than ameliorate, their general behavioral status. Some borderline patients identify the antipsychotic agents with the schizophrenic state and refuse to take them, claiming they are "not schizophrenic" and do not need "drugs for schizophrenia." In the event such drugs are tolerated, small amounts are the rule. Sedating antipsychotic agents should be avoided. Most borderline patients will not consent to depot antipsychotic drugs unless frequent and marked decompensations exist; in such cases, the diagnosis may warrant change to that of a schizophrenic illness.

The treatment of borderline patients differs from the treatment of paranoid patients in the sense that paranoid individuals are more concerned with hypervigilance while borderline individuals are concerned about problems of fusion and depersonalization. The borderline patient's symptoms often result from an inability to distinguish fantasy from fact. The physician must allay anxieties about bodily changes due to medication and the effects of medication must be spelled out in detail. Such an endeavor is bound to sensitize the patient to all medications, but the alternative is non-compliance. Borderline patients who feel their bodies to be heavier or "different" need to be asked in specific detail the nature of such sensations in order to determine whether or not it might be induced by medication or whether they simply attribute it to a drug. In fact, medication may be lessening the frequency and intensity of existing depersonalization phenomena.

Attention will now be directed to the depressive element in the borderline personality. A further discussion of this topic will be found in the next chapter pertaining to affective disorders. Changing moods seen in borderline patients often prompt clinicians to prescribe antidepressants for despondencies which are rather precipitous in onset and do not appear to have a clear basis. Antipsychotic drugs are also used in an attempt to stabilize mood much as they would be used to regulate the lability of certain schizophrenic patients. However, such mood changes and lability are characteristic of a borderline personality organization and depression should be tolerated within the limits of what is comfortable for the patient and safe for him as well. On occasion, regular clinical dosages of antidepressants are indicated although it should be recalled that such medications can activate a psychosis. Also, the side-effects of these drugs, like those of antipsychotic drugs, may be unacceptable

The depression that one sees in borderline patients is more often the manifestation of an inner emptiness that betrays the deprivations such patients incurred in early years. The despondencies are anaclitic in quality and quite haunting; no pharmacologic agent takes away this feeling and the clinician must decide whether the sadness is a genuine depression responsive to medication or simply the revelation of the patient's inner despair. The task is made more difficult because the chronic depression in these patients has both a vegetative component to it and contains elements of psychotic decompensation. Such patients do not sleep well and dislike the night when they are alone. There may be early morning awakening with anxiety and panic. Or, they may sleep too much and regressively withdraw from the world. Eating patterns may reflect anorexia nervosa-like attitudes or the disdain for food or the use of too much food. Anergia and anhedonia may prevail. All these manifestations may make the clinician reach quickly for a pill and countertransference attitudes of rescue can play a role in hastily prescribing drugs which may be either inefficacious or worsen, rather than improve, the clinical situation. It is more reasonable to look upon a significant depressive decompensation in a borderline personality as a time when psychotherapy of a more intensive nature is warranted or hospitalization should be considered.

Drug compliance in borderline patients is problematic. Borderline patients may at times become overwhelmed by their affective states of rage, anxiety, and despondency and take an overdose of medication in an attempt to quench that painful affective condition. This is not necessarily a suicidal gesture but represents aberrant thinking that more medication will simply do the job faster and more powerfully. The immediacy of demands is a core difficulty requiring the bulk of psychotherapeutic efforts. This is a far more complex matter than simply telling patients that overdoses are dangerous, a fact they already know and flaunt in crises when rescue fantasies occur. Of course, some patients take overdoses of medication in times of stress in a more consciously manipulative fashion so that this parameter needs to be addressed also.

The orality of the borderline personality is a visible trait. These patients are hungry for attention and are insatiable in their requests for affection and warmth although they are unable to tolerate the intimacy conducive to the fulfillment of these needs. Concerns about merging and fusion, or, conversely, alarm about the abandonment of close relationships leads these patients to seek transient closeness through brief encounters and promiscuity. The need for nurturance can become coupled with a pervasive quest for gratification which plays a role in attitudes towards medication. Some of these patients demand all kinds of medication, yet are frightened by vulnerabilities inherent in the transaction of compliance.

Not all borderline patients are alike, and some are extremely bothered by medications while others may have what can be labeled as addictive traits. The phenomenology of this difference is not clearly understood. Apparently, the very same impaired ego which is overwhelmed by the altered sensations resulting from medication may, in other individuals, result in a craving for pharmacologic numbing induced by alcohol, narcotics, or other medications with addictive potential. The differentiation of two kinds of borderline patients has implications for the clinician who considers medication. It may be prudent to avoid giving medications of, say, the benzodiazepine class (Librium, Valium, Serax, Lorazepam) to such patients because of concern of abuse.

It may appear paradoxical that a patient who has so many problems tolerating prescription drugs given by a clinician will seek outside drugs on the street as was the case in the above clinical example. This has in part to do with issues of control and fear of subordination to and dependence on the physician. It also relates to peer pressures and social experience of obtaining street drugs as well as the need for some disinhibition in order to acquire preliminary contact with other people. In some instances, the patient experiments with a street drug and finds the alterations in sensorium so overwhelming that a psychosis does break through. This is particularly true with hallucinogenic drugs but can occur even with the smoking of marijuana or excessive alcohol. The therapist must be aware of the patient's propensity to use illegal drugs. Such use may indicate the need for antipsychotic agents in order to protect the patient from risks of decompensation. The idea of prophylaxis is a complex one and must be presented to the patient in a straightforward manner. The clinician can tell the patient that he realizes the latter will be using drugs on the street and that,this is unfortunate but represents his desire to find a state of mind free from certain anxieties. While psychotherapy will hopefully in time identify these anxieties, medication may be useful in the interim. This message is inherently a double one in that it sanctions illicit drug use. Yet it is naive to forbid such use, and many patients justifiably complain that they have difficulty finding friends who are "clean." The message acknowledges human needs; until a therapeutic alliance is formed, borderline patients will do what they want with drugs anyway. The most that the therapist can hope for is that they take, say, a nocturnal dose of an antipsychotic drug if they are the type prone to start drug abuse.

The borderline patient may shop for prescribed or illegal drugs and discard them much as he looks for emotional attachments in life. Durable emotional investments are seen as precarious due to the possibility of disappointments. Drugs, likewise, are seen as immediate answers to problems and are promptly relinquished or discarded as they fall short of inducing states of well-being. The clinician must recognize this principle and come to grips with his own helplessness. When he sees that the patient acts as just described he must also point out helplessness to the patient in the long process required to treat these individuals. No drug is perfect for borderline patients. When drugs are used, one should be chosen and given a very adequate trial. If it is at all promising, it should be adhered to. The rule for the treatment of borderline patients is one drug, one therapist. This rule reflects the unconscious tendency toward fusion in these patients and a tendency to view the drug and the doctor as one and the same. Object stability and constancy are the utmost requirements in therapy. Familiarity and continuity supervene over any subtleties involved in changing from one drug to another.

The next case illustrates further aspects of therapy of borderline patients.

> A 43-year-old office worker was referred for psychiatric treatment because of temper outbursts and suspiciousness.
> The patient presented as a paranoid personality prone to irritability and constant jealousy regarding other workers in her office. In group therapy, she took things very personally and was constantly accusatory and verbally belligerent. A variety of clinicians had diagnosed her as

borderline on the basis of her mistrust, poor object relations, and generally demanding nature. Other personality traits were her narcissism and obsessive-compulsive traits.

Trifluoperazine 5 mg b.i.d. was prescribed for her. The patient often took this medication in moments of stress but alternately refused to take it, claiming that she "did not need" any medication and was sufficiently strong to "take on the opposition" without drugs.

This is an example of an individual who used her antipsychotic medication p.r.n. and disliked reliance upon any drug, particularly reflective of her obsessive-compulsive nature. Like paranoid patients, obsessive individuals may react to medications with disdain and a wish to "do it themselves." Nevertheless, it was markedly evident to all observers when the above patient was not on medication. On medication she behaved with much less mood lability and demonstrated less of an accusatory demeanor. She was productive in group therapy sessions and was able to make useful comments. When not taking medication, the patient was defiant, hostile, and chronically suspicious. Despite full knowledge of the benefits of medication as conveyed to her by group members, her clinicians, and her husband and family, the patient adamantly used the medication as a weapon and defensively employed it to ward off full compliance with any psychotherapeutic or pharmacologic regimen. This patient illustrates another problem relating to fear of passivity and subjugation by the doctor. In the above case, the patient remained "untouchable" and no one could control her. She was supremely dominant over any therapist and group member and defied all attempts at tractability. Many patients refuse drugs with full knowledge of the capacity of such drugs to improve their mental state. This patient became enraged when other people told her to "take your medication," a regressive comment that made her feel "like a child." Yet she inevitably generated such comments by her behavior and invited the deprecatory remarks which gave fuel to her narcissistic and paranoid posture of disdain.

The only solution for patients with this problem is to acknowledge a posture of defeat. The therapist can state that the patient seems to wish pharmacologic autonomy despite knowledge of possible benefit derived from the regular ingestion of some medication. The most a clinician can do is to say that he is of the opinion that maintenance medication may be useful and that the patient himself must decide upon compliance. Again, as with the paranoid, such a stance gives maneuvering room to patients who might otherwise entirely throw over a psychotherapeutic involvement. The issue of trust can also be acknowledged; patients can be told that both parties mistrust each other to some degree but will try to work toward a day when they can do away with such mistrust. It should also be pointed out that mistrust pervades all aspects of the patient's life and it is not limited to medication or therapy. This being the case, the world must be an unpleasant place to live in. Medications may ease some burdens but not alleviate all pain. Knowledge of the limitations of medication may be conducive to discussion about other disappointments in the patient's life.

The use of depot antipsychotic medication is exemplified by the next case example.

> A 35-year-old office worker was hospitalized on several occasions because of boisterous and belligerent behavior, grandiosity, and looseness of associations and tangential thinking. On previous occasions she had taken an array of antipsychotic medications and had been tried unsuccessfully on lithium. Her compliance was poor and she generally did not adhere to any pharmacologic regimen. She was diagnosed as being schizophrenic, schizoaffective type. She was eventually placed on depot fluphenazine decanoate, 25 mg every 2 weeks. This medication was eventually given to her every 6 weeks and the patient showed a stable outpatient course the ensuing 2½ years.

This patient illustrates several aspects of the treatment of psychoses. First, she demonstrates the utility of depot antipsychotic drugs which are recognized as being useful agents for patients troubled by compliance problems. Depot preparations offer the additional advantage of low milligram dosages even when compared with high potency oral antipsychotic agents. Thus 25 mg of fluphenazine decanoate given over a 2-week period was as effective as 700 mg of the oral form given over the same period of time. It has been suggested that the potency of depot preparations is due to the fact that these drugs are absorbed into the blood and pass directly to the brain before reaching the liver, thereby avoiding hepatic deactivation (13). Therefore, a much higher level of drug may be made available to the central nervous system than would be achieved by oral administration. The fact that low doses are used may be responsible for the low incidence of tardive dyskinesias seen in patients receiving depot preparations. Other toxicities such as those affecting the hepatic and hematopoietic systems are also very rare.

Generally, there are several indications for the use of depot preparations. The first indication would be for patients with poor compliance or those at risk who have demonstrated failure to adhere to oral regimens. A second indication may be patients who absorb oral psychotic agents poorly. In working with chlorpromazine, some workers have identified patients who have lower plasma levels than would be expected following oral dosages (37). In these patients, the difference appeared to be in gastric malabsorption or deactivation. Thus, patients who do not respond clinically to adequate oral dosages of antipsychotic medication may be absorbing the drug poorly, assuming that they are taking their medication to begin with. Parenteral dosages of the same drug may shed light on this process. If clinical response follows limited parenteral use, consideration of a depot preparation is indicated.

Another factor which should be considered in patients with inadequate responses to oral medication is the interaction between antipsychotic agents and antiparkinsonian agents. Antiparkinsonian agents may lower the antipsychotic plasma levels. The exact mechanism of such interference is unknown and thought to relate to hepatic enzyme deactivation or gastric inhibition. The clinician should thus consider withdrawing antiparkinsonian medication in patients who are not responding to adequate oral antipsychotic drugs.

Recent pharmacokinetic literature on antipsychotic drugs has shown limited correlation between clinical efficacy and plasma drug level. The state of the art here is in the early stages and made complex by the existence of varying assay techniques for the differing metabolites of these drugs (27); in some studies, patients with low blood levels have shown to be poor clinical responders while those with moderate dosages were good responders and those with high levels demonstrated toxic responses. There has also been noted an occasional patient with an adequate blood level who does not respond to the drug. Such a phenomenon can be seen with anticonvulsants also. The relevance of this for the clinician lies in the need to question drug effectiveness in the absence of clinical improvement; an alternate class or preparation of antipsychotic drug should be considered.

Depot preparations have been used by endocrinologists for years but their use in psychiatry is more recent. Many clinicians are loathe to use depot preparations for fear that the drug will be "in the system" and cannot be removed should a toxic reaction occur. This fear is often coupled with the erroneous perception that neurologic reactions from parenteral medications are worse than those from oral medications. As previously mentioned, such reactions are not necessarily more severe but occur more quickly, thus giving the illusion of severity. Reactions to depot preparations can be handled with antiparkinsonian drugs and conservatism in initial dosages should mitigate against severe adverse reactions in the early phases of drug administration.

With regard to the depot drug being "in the system," it should be noted that once the body is impregnated with an oral antipsychotic agent, that drug cannot be removed any more quickly than if the same depot substance in equivalent dosage had been injected. Yet, the psychodynamics of the two situations are different. The patient receiving a depot antipsychotic medication recognizes in some manner that the drug stays in the body for several weeks and is renewed at the end of this time. The patient must then live with a certain burden; that burden relates to the fact that there is a medication reservoir within him that he cannot remove or cannot be removed by the physician. Patients receiving oral medications have control over intake of their drugs and can stop them. Even though blood levels are sustained, the fantasy of being able to control a regimen is an important aspect of control. The depot preparations can induce passivity in patients, particularly, as is the case in many clinics, when disinterested third parties administer the injections. Physicians should acquaint themselves with the gluteal injection process in the presence of attendants or nursing staff so that they become active participants in the process of using these long-acting preparations. Such activity is conducive to patient dignity.

Patients having received no previous phenothiazine medication may be given oral fluphenazine medication to determine response and tolerance (7). After an adequate trial, the patient can be then switched to the depot form. Dose comparability between oral and depot is unknown. Thus, initial dosage of depot drugs should be conservative. If the patient has a history of having developed a neurologic reaction to an antipsychotic agent, he can be given a test intramuscular dose of 0.1 ml. If tolerated, 0.5 ml can be given during the 2nd week, and 1 ml can be given during the 3rd week. For many patients, full dosage can begin immediately. The patient in the above case example was given the depot drug in what is considered to be a standard beginning dose. There is some difference between decanoate and enanthate forms of the drug; the former has a somewhat longer span of action of 2 to 3 weeks while the enanthate has a mean length of action of 2 weeks. More conservative dosages are used with the decanoate form of the drug.

As in all antipsychotic drugs, maintenance involves giving lower dosages over greater lengths of time. For example, maintenance might be achieved by giving as little as 0.1 ml (2.5 mg) of the depot drug over a 6-week period.

Depressive mood changes have been described in association with depot fluphenazine use (1). It must be recognized that any antipsychotic agent has depressant properties. More important, however, is the fact that the pharmacologic abolition of a psychosis confronts the patient with reality as the latter becomes aware of his diagnosis and the nature of his psychotic defenses. Depot preparations probably induce depression no more frequently than oral medications do. Depression is a common finding among schizophrenic patients who are treated (32). In fact, some psychotherapists find depression a useful prognostic sign indicating that the patient is coming to grips with the relinquishment of his thought disorder. It is useful for a patient to grieve over his psychosis; a patient who goes directly from psychosis to non-psychosis without awareness of his illness is lacking in a certain insight which has potential adaptive value in the prophylaxis of future psychotic episodes.

In the case of the patient in the most recent case example, a clinician interviewed her 2 years after she had been attending a drug clinic and asked her why she had not yet returned to work. She replied that she still felt ashamed of her illness, chronically depressed, and fearful of the exacting nature of her work. This knowledge was obtained late in the course of aftercare and reflects the fact that perceptions of patients in drug clinics are often based upon observable behavior only. Residual components of psychotic illnesses such as shame, guilt, and despondency are often present and must be elicited and dealt with in some form of psychotherapy. Clinicians are often loathe to query the patient about finer functioning for fear of discovering existing psychopathology that takes time to correct. Regrettably, no cure from psychotic illness is perfect and years of recovery are the rule, not the exception.

Three complex cases will now be presented to illustrate the rational and irrational use of antipsychotic agents. These cases come from maintenance drug clinics and represent the cumulative errors made by clinicians who rotate through such facilities and often become oriented toward the simple dispensing of medication. However, these errors can occur in private practice as well.

> A 54-year-old woman was seen in a clinic because of "nerves." The patient revealed a past history of several hospitalizations because of hallucinations which told her about all her friends who were dead. When seen, she demonstrated loose associations and some anxiety as she described these hallucinations. There was no evidence of paranoid ideation and her mood appeared somewhat flat in view of the content of her hallucinations. A diagnosis of schizophrenia of a chronic type was made and the patient was placed on thioridazine, 50 mg a.m. and 100 mg h.s. She became quite drowsy on this medication and the dose was reduced to 50 mg h.s. Although it was noted that she was markedly improved during her subsequent monthly visits to the clinic and that she displayed no delusions or hallucinations, the medication was maintained for approximately 8 months at which time she was switched to thiothixene 2 mg t.i.d. because of weight gain; this dose was eventually decreased to 2 mg b.i.d. Approximately 1 year after her initial clinic visit, she was thought to be despondent and placed on amitriptyline (Elavil) 25 mg b.i.d. and 50 mg h.s. This medication was prescribed in conjunction with the thiothixene.

This case illustrates several issues in the treatment of psychoses. The patient's medication regimen was irrational. Few patients could have adhered to the complex prescriptions and there was no reason not to consolidate medications into single nocturnal dosages.

Patients on several drugs such as the above case should be asked to "brown bag" all existing drugs they have and use, including such items as vitamins or "heart pills." It is often surprising to discover the array of pharmacologic agents the patient is being exposed to.

The patient was initially diagnosed as having a chronic schizophrenic illness and given thioridazine medication which made her lethargic. This is not surprising, considering the fact that this phenothiazine is one of the more sedating drugs. In this case, the patient was taken off the drug because of weight gain and switched to thiothixene, a drug with a lower milligram daily dosage. This move may have been warranted since low potency drugs requiring high milligram dosages may produce greater degrees of weight gain. Weight gain is problematic among patients on antipsychotic medication (20). Attention must be addressed to it and careful dieting and exercise are the safest form of treatment. Certain anorectic drugs with central nervous system stimulating properties have been ineffectively used to suppress appetite;

these are contraindicated because they may exacerbate a psychosis. Weight and body image are problematic for many schizophrenic patients. Traditional psychodynamic formulations have equated weight gain with remissions from psychosis and weight loss with exacerbation; the less obese and more attractive a patient becomes, the greater is the chance for intimacy. Thus, the patient is apt to use psychotic defenses when opportunities for closeness become greater. These dynamics may be operative in any particular patient and should be explored.

During one visit to the clinic, a new therapist felt the patient to be despondent and added amitriptyline to the regimen. Such additions of antidepressant medication are not unusual in the treatment of schizophrenia and may at times be warranted. However, it is necessary that akinesia be ruled out as a condition which closely mimics despondency in chronic schizophrenic patients. The akinesia may manifest itself in psychomotor retardation, fixed and immobile facies, and general lethargy which make the patient appear to be depressed. An antiparkinsonian drug should be tried to test this hypotheses. Should the patient's mood continue to be one of true despondency, the clinician can consider a less sedating antidepressant such as imipramine (Tofranil) particularly if fatigue or inertia has been a clinical problem. The flattened affect of the schizophrenic should always enter into the differential diagnosis.

Despondencies often occur as a reactive condition to stresses at home. Such stresses are often not asked about in clinic settings. Chronically ill schizophrenic patients are not immune to mood alterations and are surprisingly sensitive to changes in the environment, including the physician whom they see only a few times a year.

Mood changes are frequently seen in chronically institutionalized patients also. Here the clinician is faced with diagnostic decisions about organic brain syndromes, endocrine abnormalities such as hypothyroidism, neurologic complications previously described, or functional affective disorders. More often than not, little can be found diagnostically. Most dismaying is the anergy, anhedonia, and apathy shown by many chronic schizophrenic patients. Some clinicians refer to this as the "burning out" process of schizophrenia, and it is commonly seen in maintenance clinics as well as institutions. Family and friends ask that the patient be given new medication or somehow be activated when in reality there may be little that can be done. Schizophrenia is an illness which leaves its residual mark upon the patient. The "burned out" schizophrenic is a clinical problem. Often such patients are kept on maintenance medication when none is justified; the development of a tardive dyskinesia may be more socially disabling than the primary illness. Attempts to withdraw antipsychotic drugs should be made. After akinesia is ruled out, antiparkinsonian agents should also be withdrawn. Often, seeing a patient in the drug-free state will reveal him to be less disabled than might be thought.

The clinician asked to see such patients should take a thorough drug history, establish that medications have been used in adequate dosages, rule out organicity, the toxic effects of existing drugs, and assure himself that there are no target symptoms that are drug responsive. When there is affect, particularly in response to delusions and hallucinations and where the patient responds with excitation or even anger and agitation to the voices he hears and the misperceptions he senses, there is hope for pharmacologic control. It is when the patient placidly accepts a hallucination without any affective response that the clinical picture and prognosis becomes bleak. At this point, in severe cases where the clinical picture is rather hopeless, unusual remedies may be attempted. A careful pondering of risk/benefit ratio is necessary should the clinician try more unorthodox means of treating such patients with antidepressants, electroconvulsive therapy, or central nervous system stimulants. Some workers have reported on the use of very large "megadoses" of antipsychotic drugs to treat refractory patients; such use should be considered experimental (36).

Rather strong countertransference sentiments are evoked by these kinds of patients. Helplessness is a common feeling in the clinician who comes in contact with such schizophrenics and there is a tendency to switch medications to avert such sentiments or to increase dosages in the act of doing something rather than nothing. While zealousness is commendable, the clinician must be in touch with his own affect and recognize that there are patients for whom one does exhaust all avenues of somatic therapy. Anger, as well as helplessness, may also be mobilized by these patients. Mental health staff may refer to such a patient in a pejorative way as a "chronic schiz." The term has connotations indicating that the patient is a zombie and devoid of human qualities. The anger also betrays the fact that clinicians are rarely acknowledged as healers by these patients. Patients with affective disorders such as depression or anxiety are generally thankful for therapeutic intervention. Psychotic patients rarely show the same degree of gratitude. In part, this stems from the fact that the clinician is taking away from such a patient an illness which has adaptive and defensive value. Another part of the lack of appreciation is inherent in the thought disorder itself and relates to the limited affective repertoire of the patient who is often insensitive to those around him and shallow in his emotional responses.

In the absence of pharmacologic improvement, many chronic schizophrenic patients can be integrated into society in some sheltered environment and even rehabilitated through intensive social input. Regrettably, this is far more difficult to carry out than rendering of drugs. Institutionalization and custodial care is more easily furnished than the teaching of rudimentary skills which would make such patients somewhat productive members of society. Families, also, show varying degrees of willingness to work with patients. Even when the family ostensibly incorporates the psychotic patient into its midst, emotions run so high and the atmosphere is so heavily charged that the patient might be better off in a more neutral environment. When the clinician is using antipsychotic drugs, he should be aware of the fact that drug needs reflect family pressures. Increasing the dose is not nearly as effective as intervening in the family since the latter can always sabotage pharmacologic control.

The role of the milieu in the treatment of psychoses has always received attention in the literature. Some clinicians have advocated the milieu as an effective modality of treatment which frees the patient from any hazard of drug use and represents a dignified cure (12). Reports of remission within the structure of a milieu should induce the psychopharmacologist to be humble and recognize that certain psychotic patients benefit solely from social structure. However, a psychosis is generally a highly unpleasant affective state and is retrospectively recalled as such by patients who remember the perplexity, loss of control, or frightening delusions. This fact forms a basis for prompt pharmacologic control, even though treatment takes away an opportunity to observe psychotic process in a natural state. While such investigation of a psychosis could be carried out during the time that the patient is actively ill, it is probably more humane to engage in this matter in therapy after improvement despite the fact that much of the content is obviously repressed as a process of cure. The point to be made is that medication should not preclude later exploration of the illness for the dynamics of a psychosis are a clue to the patient's vulnerability for relapse and should never be dismissed.

> A 32-year-old man developed a paranoid psychosis during which he felt his wife was unfaithful to him and in collusion with the FBI and CIA. He assaulted her. He was hospitalized and ultimately received 500 mg a day of chlorpromazine, 30 mg a day of trifluoperazine, 4 mg of benztropine mesylate a day, and a benzodiazepine for sleep. He had been receiving the same antipsychotic regimen for three years. The patient's only spontaneous complaint was he had insomnia and a dry mouth.
>
> On mental status, the patient showed psychomotor retardation with flat affect, immobile facial expression, and despondency. He replied, on questioning, that he had no ambition and did not wish to look for work. He denied delusions or hallucinations and there was no obvious suspiciousness.

This case example illustrates further principles in the maintenance management process. The patient was receiving two antipsychotic agents given him without clear rationale. The patient seemed lethargic and showed the mask-like facies of parkinsonism and the psychomotor retardation associated with this condition. Cogwheeling of his extremities was noted on physical examination. When elicited, he complained about muscle stiffness.

There are several possibilities to be considered in this case. It was obvious that the patient was oversedated and that he was receiving too much antipsychotic medication. Certainly, one drug would be preferable for maintenance and that would be the drug with the highest potency per milligram. It was decided to discontinue the chlorpromazine since the incidence of all long-term side-effects seem more prominent with this type of medication.

The existence of neurologic signs could be explained by the combination of chlorpromazine and trifluoperazine. The antiparkinsonian drug had limited effects on the extrapyramidal reactions despite adequacy of the dose. Indeed, upward titration of the latter drug might summate with the anticholinergic properties of the existing antipsychotic agents and produce an atropine-like psychosis. The cumulative anticholinergic effects might be responsible for the dry mouth which this patient found particularly troublesome. Generally, it appeared as though all adverse reactions might be decreased by the discontinuation of chlorpromazine and a reduction in trifluoperazine to the lowest maintenance level needed to prevent relapses. Actually, the patient had never experienced a discontinuation of his maintenance medication or reduction so that his potential for relapse was unknown. Strong psychological pressures were brought to bear on the continued use of maintenance medication because of the severity of the patient's psychosis and his alarming violent behavior. Indeed, upon discontinuation of the chlorpromazine, the wife announced that she was taking the patient's child to a nursery during the day rather than leave her with the husband since she was afraid that the husband was "showing more emotion" and could again become assaultive. It became clear that the wife wanted this patient tranquilized in order to avoid the possibility of attack.

When the chlorpromazine medication was withdrawn, the patient's gait improved and he showed decreased facial rigidity. He became more cheerful and smiled. The obvious diminution in drug-induced lethargy resulted in his being somewhat more spontaneous at home with his family. Yet while the clinician felt enthusiastic about this subtle change, the wife viewed it with alarm. In time, she might well have exerted some negative effect on the patient's full recovery; her reactions to his improvement might exacerbate underlying paranoia.

The patient receiving antipsychotic medication for long periods of time should not be seen alone but in the presence of family members. The clinician can then view the role members play in the maintenance process and establish their attitudes toward risks attendant to withdrawal from medication. There are vulnerabilities not only for the patient who improves from a psychosis but also for the family who must deal with him. Some families would prefer to have an invalid in their midst whom they can tolerate and who can serve as a focus for other familial conflicts. Other families are healthier, more willing to be recruited into efforts of resocialization, and can be drawn into the treatment process to reduce medication needs.

The neurologic reactions induced by antipsychotic drugs have been previously mentioned in detail because they play such an integral role in clinical use. Other less obvious adverse reactions will now be discussed (40). These reactions may confuse the clinician because they are so diverse and occur in such a seemingly random fashion. However, they can be logically conceptualized as side-effects and extensions of the pharmacologic properties of the drugs, or as toxic or adverse reactions which may be idiosyncratic or allergic in nature. Side-effects usually occur early in the course of treatment and are predictable, so that the skill of managing them lies in their anticipation. Toxicities or adverse reactions can be divided into those which may occur early in therapy and those which may occur after prolonged treatment with high dosage. Toxicities are generally less expected and confront the clinician with the need for vigilance.

All antipsychotic medications have anticholinergic properties and thus produce predictable side-effects which are distinct from toxicities. The most common side-effects are dry mouth, blurred vision, and constipation. Other effects such as urinary retention, intestinal obstruction, or the exacerbation of glaucoma, are rarer and may occur in patients determined by history and review of symptoms to already be at risk. Symptomatic relief may be offered for some side-effects. Dry mouth is particularly bothersome. It is of limited duration and usually remits after a week or two of medication. In the interim, sugarless lozenges or sugarless gum may be used. The reasons for sugarless preparations relates to the absence of saliva which is conducive to the development of dental caries. Laxatives may be useful for constipation.

The cardiovascular effects of antipsychotic medications should be anticipated. They are most problematic, particuarly in older patients. Orthostatic or postural hypotension can occur rather promptly upon the introduction of these drugs and is presumed to be due to a sympathetic blocking effect. Low potency phenothiazines are most notorious for inducing hypotension; for example, chlorpromazine is one drug most often associated with reductions in blood pressure. Thioridazine additionally may produce impaired ejaculation, a troubling side-effect for adolescents and certain paranoid patients concerned with sexuality and masculinity. Thioridazine is also the drug most implicated in cardiac arrhythmias. The clinician should be alert to the possibility of hypotension when symptoms of dizziness are reported. Instructions regarding the slow movement out of bed and the progressive change from a supine to sitting to standing position is helpful; abrupt changes in posture are dangerous. Elastic stockings to reduce reservoir pooling may help with orthostatic hypotension. Particular concern should be directed to patients with coronary artery disease who may develop postural hypotension when they receive antipsychotic drugs.

Toxic or adverse reactions are less predictable. Hepatic and hematologic reactions are more apt to manifest themselves in the first 2 months of therapy; thereafter, the risk drops significantly. Thus, the clinician needs to maintain an index of suspicion during the high risk period. The next case illustrates this point.

> A 57-year-old female with a history of chloromycetin-induced agranulocytosis 10 years earlier presented with symptoms of an agitated depression. She was treated with thioridazine. Baseline and weekly complete blood count determinations were performed for the first 3 weeks. It was discovered that the patient's white cell count had dropped from 8000 to 4000; the differential count was normal. Her red cell count had decreased also.
>
> Hematologic consultation corroborated the diagnosis of a drug-related pancytopenia. All medications were discontinued, and blood values returned to normal within several weeks.

The above example illustrates the development of a blood dyscrasia which occurred 3 weeks after the onset of pharmacologic treatment. Blood dyscrasias are more likely to occur in elderly females. Because of an allergic history, the clinician was sensitive to the possibility of an adverse reaction and did obtain pretreatment blood work. The subsequent periodic hematologic studies were of dubious value and it was only fortuitous that the blood dyscrasia was detected by them. It is now recognized that blood counts have little value in detecting hematologic changes which can occur a few days after a completely normal count. Clinicians may chose to advise certain patients that reversible blood changes can occur and that they should inform the doctor if a sore throat persists or if they develop any kind of recurring infection or fever. The same principle is true for hepatic toxicity. Baseline liver profiles may be of interest in high risk groups; follow-up profiles are costly and hepatic injury can be detected by the recognition of clinical signs and symptoms. Parenthetically, in the above case, a higher potency drug might have been a preferred pharmacologic agent as the risk of hematologic toxicity was higher with the agent used.

Toxic endocrinologic disturbances may follow more prolonged treatment with antipsychotic drugs. Heat and sun intolerance are not uncommon in patients receiving these drugs. Exposure to excess sun may lead to skin reddening and patients should be counselled to take sun screen lotions when they go to the beach. Strenuous exercise should also be avoided and patients should keep cool in hot weather. The difficulties with heat loss are presumably due to hypothalmic inbalance and the absence of sweating which is often exacerbated by the combination of an antipsychotic and antiparkinsonian agent, both of which have anticholinergic properties.

Other long-term endocrine changes include galactorrhea or amenorrhea and reduction in libido in men and women. There are psychological issues surrounding these changes which must be discussed with patients since they are often not volunteered to the clinician.

With prolonged administration of certain antipsychotic agents, pigmentary changes may appear in the skin, cornea, lens, and retina. These developments are more likely in individuals receiving high dosages of low potency phenothiazines for periods of many months or years. Various workers have hypothesized that these pigmentary changes relate to blocking of melanocyte-stimulating hormones. Thus, these alterations too, can be considered endocrinologic abnormalities.

The majority of toxic reactions in organ systems are dose- and time-related. The best way to avoid them is to use high potency drugs for the shortest period possible. Drug holidays reduce cumulative dose intake.

The clinician must reassure the patient about these side-effects which are predictable and represent, in part, the fact that the drug is working. He must also alert the patient and the family about less predictable adverse reactions. The above mentioned burdens of keeping cool, needing suntan lotion, dealing with dry mouth, constipation, and needing to monitor infections are significant concerns for any patient already beset by delusions or hallucinations. Patients have vastly ambivalent feelings about medications to begin with and such feelings are not helped when they must be made to worry about the emergence of multiple toxicities and side-effects. Much reassurance is necessary. Many bodily changes are confused with the primary illness. For example, endocrine changes are often ascribed to the psychosis or residual psychotic illness. It is of relief for a patient to recognize that reductions in libido may relate to medication and be reversible rather than represent permanent sequellae of his psychiatric disease.

Side-effects and toxicities play a prominent role in the treatment of the elderly (28). Physiologic changes in geriatric patients include a generally diminished capacity for the metabolic handling of drugs. With age, blood flow is redistributed toward coronary and cerebral circulations. Thus, the liver and kidney blood flows are reduced and these functions are compromised. Gastric absorption may be impaired. In the elderly, there tends to be more fat in relation to total body weight and this produces a reservoir for the increased storage of fat-soluble drugs, including antipsychotic agents. Drugs may thus accumulate due to reduced absorption, deactivation, and excretion. Small dosages are the rule for geriatric patients. The high potency antipsychotic drugs are useful because they are less prone to produce cardiovascular reactions such as hypotension. The low dosages used make neurologic reactions less likely to occur. In rarer cases of existing neurologic diseases such as parkinsonism, low potency drugs may be cautiously given as these are associated with a low incidence of neurologic reactions.

The shunting of blood flow to the cerebral circulation is a homeostatic measure designed to maintain declining brain function in the elderly. Yet such cerebral circulation may be insufficient, and senile patients may develop organic brain syndromes with psychotic manifestations. The etiology of such organic brain syndromes needs to be determined but an antipsychotic agent, used sparingly, may be helpful in these patients.

Antiparkinsonian agents must be given very carefully to older people because of their sensitivity to the atropine-like properties of this drug.

Paranoid ideation is not uncommon in geriatric groups and leads to problems with compliance and oral intake.

Certain drug interactions need to be kept in mind. Blood pressure may be significantly reduced when antipsychotic agents are combined with diuretics or antihypertensive drugs.

Adverse reactions also shape the therapy of children. It is generally recognized that the pharmacologic treatment of childhood psychoses is less satisfactory than the treatment of the adult illness (11). Antipsychotic medication often causes sedation before any antipsychotic effect is observed. As childhood psychoses usually manifest themselves through symptoms of social withdrawal and psychomotor retardation, such lethargy is particularly troublesome since the aim of treatment is to activate the child toward social interaction. Such a push is best accomplished by vigorous psychosocial therapies and drugs are perhaps more adjunctive than is the case for adults. Medications are usually most useful when there are target symptoms of insomnia, hyperactivity, impulsivity, and aggressiveness.

Fewer organ system toxic reactions have been reported in children receiving antipsychotic medications, but this may reflect the fact that lower dosages have been used for shorter periods of time; literature in this area is small in comparison with that for adult populations. It should be recalled that children are generally less verbal than adults and cannot describe toxicities which do occur. Instead, they express untoward effects such as subtle neurologic reactions or lethargy more globally and motorically. Their responses are more nonspecific and like those associated with anything emotionally unpleasant; thus, the clinician may observe apathy, irritability, decreased frustration, tolerance, or loss of appetite. Drug effect is less predictable in children and more empirical approaches to the psychopharmacologic treatment of children may be warranted. High potency phenothiazines may have more stimulatory effect than otherwise observed with adults. Also, requirements for medication may vary more widely than for adults and it is a frequent error to underestimate a child's tolerance for antipsychotic medication and to give dosages which are ineffective. As with adults, slow titration upward is the rule.

REFERENCES

1. Alarcon, R., and Carney, M. W. P. Severe depressive mood changes following slow release intramuscular injection. Br. Med. J., 3:564–567, 1969.
2. American Psychiatric Association Task Force on Nomenclature and Statistics Diagnostic Manual of Mental Disorders III, Draft, Jan. 15, 1978.
3. Anderson, W. H., Kuehnle, J. C., and Catanzano, D. M. Rapid treatment of acute psychosis. Am. J. Psychiatry, 133:1076–1078, 1976.
4. Asnis, G. M., Leopold, M. A., Duvoisin, R. C., and Schwartz, A. H. A survey of tardive dyskinesia in psychiatric outpatients. Am. J. Psychiatry, 134:1367–1370, 1977.
5. Appleton, W. S. The snow phenomenon: Tranquilizing the assaultive. Psychiatry, 28:88–93, 1965.
6. Ayd, F. J., Jr. Neuroleptic-induced extrapyramidal reactions: Incidence, manifestations and management. In The Future of Pharmacotherapy: New Drug Delivery Systems, F. J. Ayd, Jr. (Ed.). International Drug Therapy Newsletter, Baltimore, 1973.
7. Ayd, F. J., Jr. The depot fluphenazines: A reappraisal after 10 years' clinical experience. Am. J. Psychiatry, 132:491–500, 1975.
8. Ayd, F. J., Jr. (Ed.). Ethical and legal dilemmas posed by tardive dyskinesia. International Drug Therapy Newsletter, 11:29–36, 1977.
9. Blackwell, B. Patient compliance. N. Engl. J. Med., 289:249–252, 1973.
10. Blackwell, B. Rational drug use in psychiatry. In Rational Psychopharmacotherapy and the Right to Treatment, F. J. Ayd, Jr. (Ed.). Ayd Medical Communications, Ltd., Baltimore, 1975.
11. Campbell, M. Psychopharmacology in childhood psychosis. In Recent

Advances in Child Psychopharmacology, R. Gittleman-Klein (Ed.). Human Sciences Press, New York, 1975.

12. Carpenter, W. T., Jr., McGlashan, T. H., and Strauss, J. S. The treatment of acute schizophrenia without drugs: An investigation of some current assumptions. Am. J. Psychiatry, 134:14–20, 1977.

13. Cole, J. O. Introduction: Symposia on long-acting phenothiazines in psychiatry. Dis. Nerv. Syst. 31(Suppl.):5, 1970.

14. Davis, J. M. Overview: Maintenance therapy in psychiatry: I. Schizophrenia. Am. J. Psychiatry, 132:1237–1245, 1975.

15. Denber, H. C. B. Psychodynamic effects of the drug-induced extrapyramidal reactions on ward social structure. Rev. Can. Biol., 20:631–641, 1961.

16. DiMascio, A. Dosage scheduling. In Clinical Handbook of Psychopharmacology, A. DiMascio and R. I. Shader (Eds.). Jason Aronson, New York, 1970.

17. DiMascio, A. and Demirgian, E. Antiparkinsonian drug overuse. Psychosomatics, 11:596–601, 1970.

18. DiMascio, A. and Shader, R. I. Drug administration schedules. Am. J. Psychiatry, 126:796–801, 1969.

19. Gardos, G., and Cole, J. O. Maintenance antipsychotic therapy: Is the cure worse than the disease? Am. J. Psychiatry, 133:32–36, 1976.

20. Gordon, H. L., Law, A., Hohman, K. E., and Groth, C. The problem of overweight in hospitalized psychotic patients. Psychiatr. Q., 34:69–82, 1960.

21. Greenblatt, D. J., Shader, R. I., and DiMascio, A. Extrapyramidal effects. In Psychotropic Drug Side-Effects, R. I. Shader and A. DiMascio (Eds.). Robert E. Krieger Publishing Co., New York, 1970.

22. Group for the Advancement of Psychiatry, Report No. 93. Pharmacotherapy and Psychotherapy: Paradoxes, Problems and Progress. Group for the Advancement of Psychiatry, New York, 1975.

23. Havens, L. L. Problems with the use of drugs in the psychotherapy of psychotic patients. Psychiatry, 26:289–296, 1963.

24. Havens, L. L. Some difficulties in giving schizophrenic and borderline patients medication. Psychiatry, 31:44–50, 1968.

25. Hollister, L. E. Clinical Differences Among Phenothiazines in Schizophrenics. In Phenothiazines and Structurally Related Drugs, Advances in Biochemical Psychopharmacology, Vol. 9, I. S. Forrest, C. J. Carr, and E. Usdin (Eds.). Raven Press, 1974.

26. Hollister, L. E. Polypharmacy in psychiatry: Is it necessary, good or bad? In Rational Psychopharmacotherapy and the Right to Treatment, F. J. Ayd, Jr. (Ed.). Ayd Medical Communications, Ltd., Baltimore, 1975.

27. Kane, J., Rifkin, A., Quitkin, F., and Klein, D. Antipsychotic drug blood levels and clinical outcome. In Progress in Psychiatric Drug Treatment, Vol. 2, D. F. Klein and R. Gittleman-Klein (Eds.). Brunner/Mazel, New York, 1976.

28. Karasu, T. B., and Murkofsky, C. A. Psychopharmacology of the elderly. In Geriatric Psychiatry, L. Bellack and T. B. Karasu (Eds.). Grune and Stratton, Inc., New York, 1976.

29. Klein, D. F. Psychopharmacology and the borderline patient. In Borderline States in Psychiatry, J. E. Mack (Ed.). Grune and Stratton, New York, 1975.

30. Klein, D. F. Psychotropic drugs and the regulation of behavioral activation in psychiatric illness. In Progress in Psychiatric Drug Treatment, Vol. 2, D. F. Klein and R. Gittleman-Klein (Eds.). Brunner/Mazel, New York, 1976.
31. Lion, J. R. Evaluation and Management of the Violent Patient. Charles C Thomas, Springfield, Ill., 1972.
32. McGlashan, T. H., and Carpenter, W. T. Postpsychotic depression in schizophrenia. Arch. Gen. Psychiatry, 33:231–239, 1976.
33. Ostow, M. Drugs in Psychoanalysis and Psychotherapy. Basic Books Inc., New York, 1962.
34. Physicians' Desk Reference, Medical Economics Co., Oradell, N. J., 1977.
35. Quitkin, F., Rifkin, A., Gochfeld, L., and Klein, D. F. Tardive dyskinesia: Are the first signs reversible? Am. J. Psychiatry, 134:84–87, 1977.
36. Rifkin, A., Quitkin, F., Carrillo, C., and Klein, D. F. Very high dosage fluphenazine for nonchronic treatment-refractory patients. Arch. Gen. Psychiatry, 25:398–403, 1971.
37. Rivera-Calimlin, L., Nasrallah, H., Strauss, J., and Lasagna, L. Clinical response and plasma levels: Effects of dose, dosage schedules and drug interaction on plasma chlorpromazine levels. Am. J. Psychiatry, 133:646–652, 1976.
38. Sabshin, M., and Eisen, S. B. The effects of ward tension on the quality and quantity of tranquilizer utilization. Ann. N.Y. Acad. Sci., 67:746–757, 1956.
39. Sarwer-Foner, G. J. Psychodynamics of psychotropic medication. In Clinical Handbook of Psychopharmacology, A. DiMascio and R. I. Shader (Eds.). Jason Aranson, New York, 1970.
40. Shader, R. I., and DiMascio, A. (Eds.). Psychotropic Drug Side-Effects, Williams & Wilkins, Baltimore, 1970.
41. Titration and Treatment of Acute Psychosis. Panel discussion held at American Psychiatric Association Annual Meeting, 1976. McNeil Laboratories, Inc., Fort Washington, Pa., 1976.
42. Van Putten, T. Why do schizophrenic patients refuse to take their drugs? Arch. Gen. Psychiatry, 31:67–72, 1974.

Affective Disorders

In the previous chapter on thought disorders, mention was made of the target symptoms referable to behavior. In the treatment of depression, the set of target symptoms most responsive to medication are vegetative ones and include insomnia, anorexia, weight loss, constipation, lethargy, and psychomotor retardation. Mood is often less easily identified as a target symptom since despondency can arise from a variety of circumstances and be reactive, endogenous, or characterologic. Thus, there are a variety of depressive syndromes in which sadness or unhappiness is the dysphoric state. Some of these syndromes may be responsive to antipsychotic medication and some may even be responsive to antianxiety agents. Others, longstanding, may reflect chronic dissatisfaction and be responsive only to some form of psychotherapy. Not all depression is initially verbalized as such by the patient. Boredom, apathy, or lack of enthusiasm for life may be the presenting chief complaint. Impaired self-esteem and obsessive ruminations are frequent accompaniments of depression, as are anxiety and agitation. These latter symptoms may warrant the use of antipsychotic agents. Some depressions progress from simple despondency to delusions of worthlessness and are thus also responsive to antipsychotic medications; in such cases, the delusions, as well as severe agitation are the target symptoms to treat. The treatment of depression often involves the use of both antidepressants and antipsychotic agents, complicating rationales for therapy. Maintenance treatment may involve yet another medication, namely lithium, a drug specific for the treatment of mania and useful for maintenance in bipolar illness.

Anxiety is a common component of depression. It is also a distinct entity which accompanies many psychopathologic states. Anxiety reflects itself in many target symptoms such as tension or irritability, but the problem in drug control lies more in identifying when the anxiety is pathologic rather than isolating specific symptoms. Some anxiety may be situational, while other types of anxiety may be characterologically determined. Anxiety may also be the manifestation of psychotic decompensation. The use of antianxiety agents is dictated by intensity and duration of symptoms, but value judgments on the long-term use of these drugs exist.

The discussion of depression will begin with the following illustration.

> A 24-year-old male, recently alienated from his family after an argument, became progressively withdrawn and demonstrated insomnia, anxiety, concerns about his identity, and fearfulness about leaving his apartment. He felt that others at work were laughing at him. On mental status examination, the patient demonstrated flattened affect with psychomotor retardation, despondency, and episodes of sobbing. Many of these feelings he traced back to family discord.
>
> In the hospital, he was begun on amitriptyline 100 mg b.i.d. When interviewed 6 weeks later, he showed normal psychomotor activity without any evidence of despondency. Some passivity was evident as was continued concern about his future and identity. It was learned that the patient's social functioning before his illness was only moderate.

This first example is presented as one showing the problem of determining the role of drugs in the therapy of depression. Part of the difficulty of treating depressed states stems from confusions in the terminology; since there are various ways of conceptualizing depression, drug usage may vary. In the above case, the patient was seen to be suffering from a "neurotic" depression which was apparently "reactive" in nature. That is, the patient had a fight with his family and then became melancholic as an apparent reaction to that turmoil. The despondency was evident but unaccompanied by extreme despair or suicidal ideation, or by delusions or hallucinations and therefore not labeled as "psychotic." Medication was prescribed for him despite the general opinion that "reactive" or "neurotic" depressions may be treated by psychotherapy alone. The above patient turned out to have many concerns about his future, job, career, and relationship with his wife and family. There is obviously no medication affecting these concerns and verbal therapy would appear indicated. The passivity noted 6 weeks after the use of medication could have reflected residual depression but more likely indicated that some of his depression was characterologic in nature and appeared to be intimately involved with his personality. It is not unusual to find clinical examples where deviations in affective state represent changes from a baseline which is already chronically depressed due to environmental deprivations and psychosocial difficulties. It is always necessary, therefore, for the clinician to ascertain the highest level of functioning for the patient as the state to which that individual must be returned. Generally, antidepressant medications are most useful when the deviation from the baseline is very conspicuous and when the depression itself seems to be unrelated to environmental precipitants, possessing more of an "endogenous" flavor. However, this also is not always easily ascertained since small environmental occurrences often trigger the so-called "endogenous" depressions and in such cases, profound changes in mood occur from relatively trivial events. Thus, a patient may experience a serious episode of despondency following an apparently insignificant insult by a family member, and this depression may be termed "endogenous," connoting the fact that the precipitants appeared minimal and were not the obvious cause of the melancholia.

In the above case, the indication for amitriptyline was marginal, but the drug was nonetheless used with some apparent benefit. The patient complained that he had more energy and could interact more with patients on the ward. Interestingly, he also complained that he "could not cry," a sentiment occasionally verbalized by patients receiving antidepressant medication. Such medications do induce an artificial buoyancy which does not reflect itself in any euphoric or hypomanic state, but rather makes the patient appear to be sustained "in mid-air," as it were. Patients describe the fact that they feel less depressed but appear to be in a state of suspended animation, unable to grieve or cry. The feeling of "numbness" may relate to the lethargy induced by the medication which may have been the case with amitriptyline, a tricyclic antidepressant with more sedating properties than imipramine. Nevertheless, the psychological changes induced by antidepressant medications warrant acknowledgment by clinicians.

Sometimes, more commonly, depression is such that crying does not occur until there is some improvement in psychomotor retardation which allows the patient to grieve.

Depression is often conceptualized as a disruption in cerebral pleasure and reward mechanisms or mirth responses; these alterations appear to be the cardinal features of all depressions, whether or not they are "neurotic," "psychotic," "reactive," or "endogenous." Almost all patients appear to have an inability to enjoy themselves and feel some degree of sadness or guilt. The alterations in the capacity for pleasure may remain a symptom most resistant to change by antidepressants. As is the case for thought disorders, the clinician sees first changes in psychomotor functioning with drug use. In the above case, staff remarked that the patient slept better, walked more quickly, dressed with more enthusiasm, and interacted more with patients. However, as mentioned, there still remained defective self-image with decreased interest in the outside world and a lack of capacity to achieve a full degree of zest from other people and the surroundings. Not all of these types of symptoms remit with proper dosages of antidepressant medication but respond more to psychotherapy which must be continued after symptomatic improvement. As previously mentioned, some symptoms may turn out in time to reflect personality traits resistant to change.

Of studies done to date in the efficacy of certain antidepressant medication, it has been shown that approximately 60% of depressed patients improve on antidepressant medication while 40% improve on placebo (4). This being the case, it is evident that antidepressants may have utility which is not as marked as is the case for antipsychotic drugs. Many depressions remit spontaneously and improve with simple reassurance or a therapeutic milieu; in many instances antidepressants play an adjunctive role in the treatment of depression as probably illustrated in the above example.

The following case examplifies an incident of depression for which the indication for antidepressant drugs appeared clearer, at least retrospectively.

A 59-year-old woman without any psychiatric history was self-referred with the complaint that "I have a lot of worry on me." The patient stated that she was in financial difficulty since the death of her husband. Past surgery for an orthopedic problem resulted in her being unable to do housework and the patient, over the past several months, had experienced insomnia, crying spells, and feelings of despondency. She was distraught about her arthritis and the problem of getting older. There was a history of anorexia and weight loss. Concentration and memory impairment was noted on examination. She appeared morose.

She was placed on amitriptyline medication 25 mg t.i.d. over a 3-month period. At the end of this time, the patient stated that her despondency had remitted and that she was sleeping well. She no longer felt sad and showed an improved mood and was able to do her housework.

This case illustrates a depression which was deeper and of longer duration. Her illness represented a significant deviation in baseline functioning as it was learned that her premorbid adjustment was very good. She demonstrated not only a moderately severe disturbance in mood, but also changes in cognitive abilities as well, manifested by memory impairment and difficulties in concentration. This phenomenon is not unusual in depression, where the patient is so retarded that attention is low and preoccupation high; she responded to the routine questions of a mental status examination with minimal responses. Distractibility in depression is noteworthy, and friends are often first to note that the patient is "not the same" and not as attentive as before. In some instances, work capacity is the first to suffer while in other instances, patients work longer and burden themselves with increased tasks out of a sense of guilt. When work suffers, concentration is often the root of the problem and accounts for the fact that patients will try and work even harder to cope with what situations they feel unsure of. In elderly patients, concentration impairment may reach the point of mimicking an organic brain syndrome with disorientation, perplexity, and confusion.

Associated with distractibility may be somatic preoccupation as partially illustrated by the above case. To some extent, such somatization may represent concerns about aging and death. In other instances, the patient becomes convinced that there is something seriously wrong with him and there appears to be a cognitive component to the affective disorder. On occasion, the somatic complaint assumes such magnitude that it becomes almost delusional in quality and dominates all aspects of the patient's functioning. The patient may see a malignant illness as the cause of his apathy and indifference.

The above mentioned symptoms warrant consideration of antidepressant drugs. Guidelines for the use of these medications are as follows.

As is the case with antipsychotic agents, there is no evidence that any one tricyclic antidepressant is significantly superior to existing others in terms of efficacy (24); sedating and nonsedating properties of the drugs warrant consideration in selection. Thus, amitriptyline and doxepin (Sinequan) have discernible sedative properties and may be useful for certain agitated depressions while imipramine or protriptyline (Vivactil) may be warranted in retarded depressions since they have no sedating properties. There is no evidence that the tricyclic metabolic derivatives such as nortriptyline (Aventyl) or desipramine (Pertofrane, Norpramine) are any more rapid acting or efficacious than their parent compounds.

Like the antipsychotic agents, antidepressants affect behavioral manifestations of the illness first. As mentioned, sleep returns and eating improves early and such changes can be seen within 10 days to 2 weeks. Mood, however, requires longer treatment and the clinician must be prepared to wait 4 weeks or longer to witness changes in affective state.

There is no evidence that parenteral use of existing antidepressants hastens clinical improvement. Although they are theoretically useful for patients with poor compliance, toxicities may be greater and the clinician should consider alternate treatments such as electroconvulsive therapy (ECT), to be described later. Unlike antipsychotic drugs, gastric absorption difficulties have not been described in the use of antidepressants.

Tricyclic compounds are the most commonly used class of antidepressants. They are chemical derivatives of the phenothiazine nucleus. Thus, there are predictable side-effects such as dry mouth, blurred vision, or constipation. However, antidepressants have significantly greater anticholinergic properties, resulting in the greater cardiac toxicity. Cardiac toxicity reflects itself in conduction and repolarization irregularities and arrythmias which are usually benign. However, if used in high dosages or superimposed on existing cardiac disease, such toxicities may result in serious complications. Doxepin is a tricyclic antidepressant which appears to be less associated with cardiac toxicity. However, all tricyclics can produce hypotension, necessitating particular cautions in the elderly.

The higher inherent anticholinergic properties of antidepressants results in the fact that, outside of tremor, neurologic reactions are rarely seen in clinical usage. However, titration upward must be made more cautiously than with antipsychotic agents because of cardiovascular toxicity. In the above case, a low dose of 25 mg t.i.d. was employed initially. Hypotension became apparent at 75 mg, a rather low total dose. The t.i.d. regimen was retained, rather than consolidated into one nocturnal dose which might produce greater hypotension. Divided regimens are indicated in elderly patients, or in certain patients with cardiovascular disease, particularly if the patient gets up in the middle of the night. In some cases, a ⅓ to ⅔ b.i.d. regimen is possible. In healthy individuals dosage is begun with ⅓ to ¼ of the maximum dose; this can be titrated to a maximum depending upon condition by the 2nd week. In some younger patients, the maximum dose can be given by the end of the 1st week. Like antipsychotic drugs, antidepressants have long biologic half-lives and can eventually be given in one consolidated nocturnal dose. There is no evidence that special long acting forms of antidepressants such as imipramine pamoate are more effective than the ordinary form of the drug.

Despite comments about the need for caution in the administration of antidepressants, upward titration is still indicated to the end point of demonstration of inefficacy or incipient toxicity. In fact, of all drugs used in psychiatry, antidepressants are those most often given in ineffective dosages (20). The next case illustrates this point.

A 57-year-old woman was hospitalized because of socially withdrawn behavior, unusual posturing, mutism, and profound despondency. Inappropriate behavior with giggling and accusations were noted, together with agitation. The picture was consistent with that of a psychotic depression. Imipramine 25 mg q.i.d. was begun for 1 week, but abandoned in view of a perception that a quicker response would ensue with nortriptyline. The new drug was begun in dose ranges 25 mg t.i.d. and advanced to 150 mg daily over a 5-week period. Virtually no response occurred, until the 6th week when the dose was advanced to 200 mg daily. Thereafter, complete clinical improvement occurred.

This example illustrates the lack of aggressive titration in a patient and the shifting of drug regimens. Clinicians often become disenchanted with drug response or impatient with antidepressants, or yield to the pressure of colleagues or supervisors who suggest alternate strategies of treatment as they see a depressed patient who evokes helplessness. In the above case, the dose could have been advanced faster in the absence of side-effects or toxicity to effect more rapid improvement. While a plateau of improvement is seen similar to the curve drawn by antipsychotic drugs, partial response in the absence of serious adverse reaction may justify the final increment which induces recovery. However, dosages significantly beyond those seen in the *Physicians' Desk Reference* rarely lead to major therapeutic gains and are associated with greater risks of toxicity.

Much work has been done on the relationship between plasma levels of the antidepressants and the clinical effectiveness of the drug. Much of this work is still in the investigational stage but some principles are evident (29). For most of the tricyclics, there exists a linear relationship between the dose and the therapeutic response. The one well-studied exception to this involves the drug nortriptyline (Aventyl) which produces a curvilinear dose response curve. This effect is often referred to as a "therapeutic window" because it implies that there is a critical dose range for each patient below and above which the dose will be ineffective. But the practitioner must recall that even for drugs with linear dose response characteristics, the administration of an excessive dose may be detrimental for the patient as it may produce confusion and sedation. The main practical advantage to blood level determination is the assurance of compliance on the part of the patient. Other applications include detection of non-responders who may, for example, have poor gastric absorption of the drug. It may be an advantage to determine blood levels in older patients who achieve higher blood levels at standard doses. Most commercial laboratories are currently able to perform antidepressant blood level determinations.

Recent years have witnessed the development of several new types of antidepressants, often referred to as "second generation" drugs when they are variations of tricyclic structures, or "third generation" drugs when they have unique chemical structures. Examples of the former are trimipramine (Surmontil) and amoxapine (Ascendin), while the latter group now contains a tetracyclic called maprotiline (Ludiomil) and an entirely new compound, trazadone (Desyrel). Initially touted as antidepressants with fewer side effects or possibly faster onset of action, all of these drugs have proven to be less than ideal. Most of the newer antidepressants produce cardiovascular or toxicities while others have been associated with rare but troublesome side effects such as seizures or priapism. Of the newer drugs, trazadone (Desyrel) has very low anticholinergic activity and thus may be useful in older patients who might be intolerant of the blurred vision or constipation or urinary retention attributable to this side effect. Amoxapine (Ascendin) is derived from the antipsychotic drug loxapine (Loxitane) and has been described as being of utility in the treatment of psychotic depressions. By the same token, the similarity of antidepressant to an antipsychotic drug has led to the development of neurologic reactions in some patients.

In summary, the tricyclics still dominate the therapeutic picture when it comes to familiarity of usage for the practitioner. And the principles of use with new drugs still hold: aggressive titration upward to effective dosages, patience, and a willingness to abandon the drug for another (or another modality of treatment) if the agent employed appears ineffective when tried at the right dose for the proper length of time.

One other class of drug should be mentioned in connection with antidepressant efficacy, and that is the new triazolobenzodiazepine called alprazolam (Xanax). The drug is currently marketed for "anxiety with depressive symptoms", but ongoing studies comparing it with known tricyclic antidepressants indicate that at higher dosages this drug may have a direct antidepressant effect (5). While still not appropriate for severe retarded or endogenous depressions, alprazolam (Xanax) may have utility in the therapy of milder agitated depressions with a major component of anxiety. But other benzodiazepines may also be effective with certain anxiety/depressive states, as described later on in this chapter. Thus the use of antianxiety drugs to treat agitated despondencies or characteroloic dysthymic states is not a new finding in pharmacology and represents, instead, some non-specific factors involved in the therapy of affective states. Clinicians should recall that the use of high dosages of benzodiazepines to treat depressions presents the hazard of dependency and withdrawal.

Having now discussed the use of tricyclic and some of the new classes of antidepressants, attention will be directed to an older class of drugs useful for the therapy of depression, namely the MAO inhibitors. Of the MAO inhibitors, three are currently available for use. Isocarboxazid (Marplan), trancylcypromine (Parnate), and phenelzine (Nardil) share toxicities which are quite different from the tricyclic antidepressants. Basically, all of these drugs are capable of inducing hypertensive crises when used in combination with prescribed sympathomimetic substances such as L-dopa, or epinephrine or proprietary drugs containing vasoconstrictors. In some patients, hypertensive reactions may occur upon ingestion of foods containing tryptophan and tyramine such as certain cheeses or pickled products. The MAO inhibitors must be used with caution in elderly patients or in those with existing cardiovascular disease because of effects on blood pressure. If these drugs are found to be ineffective, it is also advisable to wait several weeks before using a tricyclic drug because of interactions leading to hypertension.

In limited existing comparison studies, MAO inhibitors have been found to be less effective than tricyclic compounds (3). The pharmacologic and dietary restrictions associated with MAO drugs have made them fall in disfavor. Thus, they are considered by most clinicians as second-order choices for the treatment of depression (3, 10). Physicians are often quite frightened about the use of these drugs even though these agents may have merit in isolated cases when used with compliant patients who may be refractory to tricyclics; if personal discomfort influences the aggressiveness with which the clinician uses the drug, it is better to refer the patient to a colleague who is acquainted with the proper management and utilization of this class of drugs.

This discussion raises the issue of alternate modalities of therapy for depression, illustrated in the following example.

> A 61-year-old female was hospitalized because of depression occurring secondary to the serious illness of her husband. The patient showed diminished concentration and despondency. When admitted she demonstrated mild persecutory ideation. Her affect was flat and at times she paced. In subsequent days it was noted that she was afraid of being touched, and was often mute when spoken to. There was a question as to whether or not she was hallucinating. She ate very little and seemed unable to concentrate on ward details.
>
> The patient had been on methyldopa (Aldomet) 250 mg b.i.d.
>
> The antihypertensive medication was discontinued since it was suspected of possibly inducing depression. She was begun on imipramine 20 mg b.i.d. and this drug was titrated up to 25 mg t.i.d., but the patient became hypotensive and demonstrated EKG changes indicative of mild ischemia. Perphenazine (Trilafon) (4 mg b.i.d.) was used without any improvement. The patient eventually received ECT with a complete remission of her depression.

This case demonstrates the problem of toxicities in elderly patients. Actually, few cases pose as many problems to the clinician as the older individual with cardiac disease who suffers a depression. The need for drugs must be weighed against the risk of cardiac toxicity. In such cases, baseline EKG studies are warranted. In addition, standing and supine blood pressure readings should be taken to determine orthostatic hypotension so that titration can be more intelligently carried out. Divided dosages may be required, and low dosages at the outset are the rule. The clinician must recall that antidepressants interfere with certain antihypertensive agents such as guanethidine (Ismelin). In addition, the anticholinergic properties of these drugs can lead to an atropine-like psychosis in the elderly with compromised cerebral circulation.

In the above case, doxepin might have been considered as an alternative antidepressant. However, all drugs were abandoned and the patient was successfully treated with ECT.

Depression is a unique disease in that there exists an alternative somatic modality of therapy which is non-pharmacologic. Electroconvulsive therapy has been shown to be effective in the treatment of retarded and agitated depressions. Hence, the clinician must make a certain judgment with regard to the utilization of ECT. Need and urgency enter into this decision. Acutely suicidal patients with past histories of suicide attempts or patients with depressions and accusatory hallucinations urging them to kill themselves are high risk groups and may require ECT. Patients at risk with antidepressant drugs such as illustrated in the above case example may warrant ECT. Electroconvulsive therapy, if carefully administered, is a valuable tool. Unfortunately, the nature of the treatment is quite frightening to many patients. The sequelae of transient memory disturbance is sufficiently disturbing as to dampen the subsequent immediate usefulness of verbal psychotherapy. There is also evidence that the relapse rate from ECT is somewhat higher, necessitating longer periods of maintenance antidepressant drugs (11). Against these observations and facts must be bolstered the knowledge that there are certain patients for whom treatment is indeed an emergency and the alleviation of suffering both mandatory and humane.

Clinicians skilled in the use of ECT do probably attract patients who benefit from this procedure and perceive it as the treatment of choice. Yet other clinicians view the process of ECT with much disdain. In no area of psychiatry is there as much polarization of feeling regarding the appropriate therapy of choice for depression. The situation regarding this dicotomy is unlikely to be resolved and in part results from a complex set of variables involving patient expectation and facility with the administration of ECT. Those most prejudiced against the treatment are often inexperienced with it, while some of those highly touting the treatment often use it rather exclusively. It can only be suggested here that an open mind be maintained and that the clinician recognize that such openness is a function of the availability of choice; thus, some exposure to the use of ECT is mandatory for clinicians involved in the treatment of affective disorders and enables them to make decisions based on experience and knowledge rather than bias.

Decisions to use ECT must always take into account the patient's views and time must be spent with the patient in assessing the potential impact of the procedure on esteem as well as finer cognitive functioning. The latter is one of the most important aspects to follow in treatment.

Some depressions are so severe that they are called "psychotic." The depression reaches intolerable proportions and results in the patient's profoundly abject state. Suicidal ideation may be prominent. Additionally, there may be delusions of worthlessness and hopelessness.

> A 49-year-old woman was admitted because of depression and a recurrent fear she would harm her granddaughter.
> On admission, the patient presented as a despondent and tearful woman who described tormenting and ruminative thoughts concerning the possibility that she might be homosexual. This idea came into her mind as she thought about washing the genitals and changing the diapers of her daughter's child. In addition the patient was preoccupied with guilt about her past marriage and its failure. There was some suicidal ideation.
> She was placed on amitriptyline 200 mg h.s. and discharged as "improved" from the hospital. However, she continued to complain of the intrusion of unwanted ideas when seen as an outpatient. The dosage was titrated to 300 mg with the result that the patient stated "the thoughts sometimes come but I can make them go away." Her mood was stable. Fatigue in the morning was problematic, so the final dose was adjusted to b.i.d. regimen of 200 mg h.s. and 100 mg in the late a.m.

This case illustrates a severe depression labeled as psychotic. The depression was responsive to antidepressant medication. As with the schizophrenia, the thought disorder component resisted pharmacologic control and the patient complained of the delusional-like activity. Her initial inadequate response was due to an inadequate dose. As the dose was increased, amelioration of symptoms occurred. It would be expected that in time, the patient would make a recovery or be considered a candidate for another form of therapy to be described shortly.

Antidepressant medications must be advanced in dose to maximum in order to fully assess efficacy. Yet there are upper limits of dosage as previously described. In the above case, it is unlikely that dose ranges higher than 300 mg would have benefited the patient but would have exposed her to increased risks of toxicity.

The definition of "psychotic" depression has been problematic. Generally, as is the case with schizophrenia, delusions and hallucinations are but part of the symptoms indicative of a thought disturbance; severe devaluement of the self to the point where low esteem assumes delusional proportions is commonly seen in "psychotic" depressions. The above patient experienced the persistent intrusion of an unwanted thought which was alien, but still of a haunting nature. This was coupled with an extraordinary sense of guilt.

The delineation on a continuum from normal to psychotic depression is currently encompassed in the proposals for DSM III. Here, the clinician can grade a depression from mild to psychotic on the basis of severity. Other terms such as "involutional" or "endogenous" have been deleted.

The art in managing depressed patients depends on an understanding of the unfolding of symptomatology.

Depression leads to apathy and social withdrawal, a posture which forces the patient to become self-conscious. The self-consciousness leads to introspection which may assume obsessional proportions. As the patient repeatedly thinks about himself and his past deeds, doubts creep in about the morality and validity of actions. This, in turn, leads to more indecisiveness and ruminations. Obsessions can form the major portion of a depressive illness and be exceedingly painful, causing the patient to lie awake at night and "tape record" over and over again past faults and future difficulties. Seemingly trivial interpersonal difficulties may become insurmountable and lead the patient to perceive himself as hopeless and trapped by a variety of circumstances; remorse may be extreme. Together with these symptoms, there is a fear of loss of control and the patient will verbalize the fact that he "can't control his mind." Fears of going "crazy" or "running amok" are not uncommon. Occasional outbursts of temper may reflect intolerable ambivalent feelings which can no longer be handled by the patient. Panic may ensue. With anxiety and self-consciousness come some ideas of reference leading the patient to assume that other people must also be able to see what is wrong with him.

There are qualitative differences between the delusions of depressed patients and those harbored by schizophrenics or paranoid patients. Depressed patients generally have delusions stemming from a sense of guilt or worthlessness; the patient feels that he rightly merits punishment for past faults. Schizophrenic and paranoid patients believe that they are being harshly or unfairly treated because they have special powers; others are out to retaliate against them because of jealousy, envy, or fear. The hallucinations of depressed patients are also unlike those in schizophrenia. The depressed patient states that he may have heard voices; exploration of the content of these hallucinations will reveal that they contain derogatory comments or reflect distortions of what people have actually said.

It can be seen upon review of the depressive process that certain psychopathologic events are reminiscent of psychotic decompensation, such as obsessive ruminations with guilt. Ideas of reference and bizarre dreams and panic states indicative of a fear of loss of control are also psychotic-like in nature. With any of the above conditions may come psychomotor agitation severe enough to cause pacing, hand wringing, and constant body motion. An exaggerated sense of worthlessness may lead to delusions and hallucinations.

The cognitive disturbances seen in depression can often be identified as the primary disturbance responsible for secondary alterations in mood. Thus, the patient misperceives his errors as overwhelming and then feels despondent accordingly. This conceptualization of depression as stemming from disordered thought processes facilitates the view that antipsychotic agents may be the drugs of choice for therapy. Studies comparing antipsychotic medication such as chlorpromazine with antidepressants such as imipramine have shown that both are efficacious agents for groups of depression with cognitive disturbances and agitation (19). Panic and agitation are symptoms which shape the rationale for the use of an antipsychotic agent. Severe depressions, in fact, often have more the flavor of a psychosis then they do melancholia, despite the fact that a deep and pervasive mood change exists. The next example illustrates this.

> A 47-year-old woman was hospitalized because of withdrawn behavior, agitation, and depression. The patient maintained the conviction that people were coming into her house and that the house might catch fire although she could not elaborate on this belief. There was marked insomnia and anorexia. On examination, the patient was suspicious and uncooperative, not answering questions directly. She was markedly restless and wished to leave the interview room on many occasions. She spoke in a low tone, and acted apathetic. Her general behavior on the ward was that of profound sadness with crying.
>
> Antidepressants were begun without a change in her clinical state. She was eventually placed on haloperidol 20 mg per day which resulted in a distinct improvement allowing discharge.

In the above case, psychomotor agitation and retardation coexisted. No one could have predicted whether an antidepressant or an antipsychotic agent would help this patient. The clinician attempted the former without success, and then switched to the latter drug. He could just as well have begun the patient on antipsychotic agents, using the target symptom of agitation and the delusions as justifications for therapy.

Guidelines as to which drugs to use first are problematic. Agitated depressions may benefit from sedative antidepressants or from antipsychotic agents. Retarded depressions with delusions may also benefit from non-sedating antidepressants or antipsychotic agents. The physician is left then with choices based on the severity of psychomotor agitation and delusions and hallucinations. The best that can be said of the decision making process is that it should be guided by the clinician's perception of how severe the core mood process is and whether or not thought disorder components of the affective disorder have assumed dominance. There is some opinion to the effect that deluded depressed patients may be less responsive to antidepressants than patients without delusions (6). Thus, antipsychotic agents or even ECT may be the treatments of choice. However the issue is far from settled. It is made even more complicated by the very frequent conjoint use of both antidepressants and antipsychotic agents. Such pharmacologic mixtures are commonly used to treat depression and there exists on the market combinations of these drugs in fixed dosage forms such as Triavil (a combination of perphenazine and amitriptyline). While the use of one tablet with two components may represent a logical combination of two efficacious drugs, it is wiser to employ these drugs separately in order to monitor efficacy and toxicity. First, however, a reasonable conceptualization of the depressed state must be made to justify the rational use of any one or two psychopharmacologic agents.

In the conjoint use of antipsychotic and antidepressant medication, one drug is usually added to the second subsequent to the development of an unwanted psychopathologic condition. In the case of schizophrenia, antidepressants may be added to the antipsychotic regimen if, after prolonged use, there is evidence of a true supervening affective disturbance and akinesia has been ruled out. Conversely, antipsychotic agents may be added to an antidepressant regimen if it is observed, after time, that the patient shows signs of agitation or disordered thinking indicative of the activation of a psychosis. In certain instances, one may be justified in giving both drugs together much as one gives antiparkinsonian agents prophylactically to paranoid patients. For example, one might wish to "cover" a psychologically fragile patient having had a previous psychosis with an antipsychotic agent if that patient develops a retarded depression warranting antidepressants. The next case illustrates this point.

> A 30-year-old woman with a history of psychosis was maintained on loxapine (Loxitane) 30 mg h.s. She became depressed and showed psychomotor retardation and suicidal ideation. Protriptyline was begun at a dosage of 30 mg per day. The patient complained of bizarre and frightening dreams, together with symptoms of her body "not being right" and symptoms of depersonalization. The loxapine was increased to 50 mg with a reduction in the latter symptoms and an eventual improvement of mood.

This example demonstrates the need to monitor closely the subtle changes resulting from the use of antidepressants. A dose adjustment of antipsychotic medication was necessary in view of an apparent antidepressant toxicity manifested by symptoms indicative of an incipient psychosis. Bizarre dreams or subtle changes in body perception are often the first indicators of psychotic decompensation and can be handled by a reduction in antidepressant, or by an increase in antipsychotic medication the patient is already on. In the above case, the vulnerability of the patient to antidepressant toxicity would make consideration of antipsychotic medication mandatory in the event of future depressions should the patient, at that time, be on no such drug.

If two drugs are used concurrently from the outset, dose changes should be made with one drug at a time only. Whenever possible, the therapist must have in mind and describe on paper the reasons for adding a second drug or using two drugs. Thus, target symptoms need to be elucidated. It must be remembered that the use of an antipsychotic drug for any sustained length of time entails the risk of a neurologic reaction. The interaction resulting from antipsychotic and antidepressant agents should be kept in mind. For example, it has been shown that antipsychotic drugs can inhibit the metabolism of antidepressants (7). The conjoint use of antidepressants and antipsychotic agents may also result in more severe hypotension. Finally, the clinician must also be aware of cumulative anticholinergic properties and the atropine-like psychosis which may result from the use of two drugs.

The next case example illustrates problems of conjoint drug use.

> A 50-year-old woman was admitted because of depression following the death of her husband. She was tearful and preoccupied with the idea that in former years she had an affair with another man. She became mildly paranoid about her relatives, walked outdoors improperly clad, and showed inappropriate affect. She demonstrated psychomotor agitation and religious delusional beliefs.
>
> The patient was begun on thioridazine 50 mg b.i.d. in conjunction with amitriptyline 50 mg b.i.d. The thioridazine was increased to 50 mg q.i.d. a few days after admission. Within 1 week, the patient showed less delusional activity with more goal directed behavior. Ten days after admission, she suffered a hypotensive episode at which time she was noted to have orthostatic hypotension. The thioridazine medication was reduced to 50 mg h.s. On this regimen, she made an uneventful recovery. The antidepressant was discontinued.

In this case, several errors are demonstrated despite the fact that the patient improved. The occurrence of orthostatic hypotension may have reflected the combined use of thioridazine and amitriptyline, a particularly cardiotoxic combination. Unfortunately, there was no baseline documentation of any orthostatic hypotension, a condition not uncommon in the elderly. Knowledge of this might have influenced both choice of drug and aggressiveness of drug titration.

The clinician in this case elected to discontinue the amitriptyline following improvement, feeling that the patient's rapid symptomatic improvement was due to the antipsychotic medication rather than the low dose of antidepressant. In retrospect, the rationale for using both drugs remained unclear.

Medicating depressed patients requires verbal instructions. Since depression takes time to remit, the patient must be instructed that change will be forthcoming but that some time will be necessary for complete recovery to ensue. This mitigates against expectations of rapid recovery. Patients can be informed that the medication itself will help them sleep and eat better while their mood is being restored. Sometimes mild toxicities can be capitalized upon. The patient can be reassured that the medication is "in his system" and that improvement will follow. Relatives must also be told the course of recovery. Both patient and family also need to be appraised of the fact that there exist a variety of medications and modalities of treatment for depression and if one medication does not prove efficacious, another can be substituted in its place. Many patients in states of despondency view the psychopharmacologic process as unitary; that is, they think that there is only one drug in existence which will either help them or prove ineffective and thus doom them to a state of hopelessness.

Some statements about treatment are problematic. If ECT is mentioned as an alternative treatment, it may be perceived as more severe or drastic or as that form of therapy for those who "do not make it." The patient must be appraised of the fact that certain modalities of treatment are more efficacious for some types of depression; this does not represent the fact that he is sicker or less amenable to help.

The families of depressed patients need to be worked with in psychotherapy. Families often carry tremendous burdens during the period of depression. Husbands must work as well as take care of a spouse who is ill while wives must deal with a previously hard working husband who now sinks into abject despair and remains around the house all day long. Marital stresses inevitably ensue, particularly over the specific symptom of indecisiveness. This trait is most noxious to the families of depressed patients. Not only does the depressed patient blame himself for his own faults, but he also cannot make decisions. The helplessness evoked in others becomes intolerable. Physicians, also, are vulnerable to this dynamic and may overprescribe medications rather than listen to accounts of the indecisiveness, something which would ultimately cause the patient to have more faith in the clinician's willingness to accept him.

The families of depressed patients can, to some extent, understand depressive illness provided that the mood does not last too long. Eventually, however, they become very angry and make comments to the effect that patients should "snap out of it," or "shape up." Suicidal ideation, likewise, is frightening to families and leads them to make concrete suggestions about the value of life, a statement which has little worth in the mind of a depressed patient. The need for simple ventilation is mandatory in the case of families. Clinicians often do not wish to see the spouses of members they are treating in therapy in order to preserve confidentiality. While adhering to the policy of privacy, it is a great help to the patient and his spouse when a conjoint session is allowed to take place. Furthermore, it would seem only reasonable and humane to allow the spouse of a depressed patient to verbalize some of his feelings and ask questions of the physician regarding the course of the illness and treatment. If the therapist has strong feelings that such a move might jeopardize treatment, then he can at least consider referring the spouse elsewhere.

When depression does eventually remit, there is often an outpouring of anger on the part of spouses or other family members who have been victim to the patient's depression and have had to take up the slack during this time. Before the improvement, relatives were afraid to ventilate these sentiments lest the patient become worse. Joint sessions with the family may ease communication in this regard.

The clinician's posture in depression is important. Generally, even in analytically oriented treatment, a fairly nurturant stance is useful (25). Loss and deprivation are cardinal dynamic themes in depression. The therapist may elect to assume a dominant position in therapy, the authoritative role of a healer. Since the patient yearns to be taken care of, symptomatic amelioration may ensue. However, irrational needs are inevitably felt by the patient. As the limitations of the therapist become perceived, depression ensues. Most of this is reflected in a transference process and may be amenable to insight. Anger at the therapist, as well as at other loved ones in the patient's life, may appear. The therapist understands the genesis of anger as reflective of but one side of the ambivalence which characterizes the patient's attitude toward close object relations. Relatives and family members, however, do usually not appreciate this hostility and hardly view it as healthy. If they have spent inordinate efforts trying to help the depressed patient through his illness, they often become mystified and dismayed and translate these emotions into requests for additional medication. The clinician must explain that the anger is a time-limited phenomenon associated with recovery.

The transference process also shapes the patient's reaction to the medication. If it is positive, the patient is eager to respond to the medication and a positive placebo effect will occur. If the transference is negative, the patient is apt to be suspicious of the medication, develop many of the side-effects so prevalent with the antidepressants, and resist the proper use of the medication.

Many psychological factors play a role in the recovery from illnesses identified as depression. These factors will now be discussed in the context of several case examples.

A 56-year-old female outpatient was seen because of "nervousness" and despondency. She was a passive and dependent woman who was overweight and tended to lead a seclusive and anhedonic life. The patient came from a low socioeconomic background and her symptoms were seen as basically situational with superimposed characterologic difficulties. Chlordiazepoxide was prescribed. The patient related well to her physician through supportive therapy. In time, a new physician took over her case and noted despondency, anorexia, and agitation. She was prescribed amitriptyline in dosages ranging from 75 to 200 mg per day. She was maintained on this medication for over a year, complaining during clinic visits of "feeling blue" and social isolation.

This is a complex case, illustrating several principles relevant to the management of socially isolated and chronically depressed patients. The patient initially benefited from the supportive treatments given her by a physician with whom she had good rapport. The new clinic physician perceived a diagnosis of depression, and accordingly gave her antidepressants, a behavior which in turn appeared to shape her behavior of despondency and perpetuated the medication beyond what was reasonable. The patient had none of the vegetative signs responsive to antidepressants. Indeed, it appeared quite unnecessary for her to receive this medication which only proved to be the currency of care. Most likely, sadness on the part of the patient who missed her old doctor was identified as depression requiring pharmacologic therapy. Acknowledgment of the loss might have been more productive.

The concept of medication as the token for concern on the part of the physician has been mentioned in a previous chapter with respect to antipsychotic medication. In the area of depression, medication assumes even more of a psychological value. Patients who are isolated, lonely, or physically ill often do show sadness which, while marked, does not represent a true indication for antidepressant medication. Unfortunately, the helplessness evoked by these patients leads to improper prescriptions of antidepressant drugs. These drugs are often continued for a surprisingly long time and held in some value by the patient. While both antipsychotic and antidepressant medications induce no dependency, patients often have a surprising need for their drugs and see them as quite beneficial. In the case example above, the patient stated that she "always felt better when I took my pill in the morning." It is unlikely that this comment had a pharmacologic basis unless one considered the sedation which came about as a result of the ingestion of the drug. More likely, the patient was describing a placebo effect from the medication.

Chronic depression is also a commonly seen phenomenon. Patients with characterologically ingrained depression are misanthropic and anhedonic. They require much nurturance and have the propensity, as do certain borderline patients, for evoking this need among clinicians who can find themselves exhausted by such individuals and dread their arrival in the office. It must be recalled that the misery of chronically depressed patients keeps others at bay and serves as a defensive maneuver to avoid intimacy (10).Recognizing this principle will alleviate much anguish on the part of the doctor who must realize that certain patients will always be despondent and cannot be brought back to any semblance of happiness since their baseline state was never one containing much joy.

Group therapy with an orientation on socialization may, for a patient such as described in the recent case example, improve mood and decrease demands on the physician's time. Certain patients are able, through intensive psychotherapeutic work, to recognize this capacity they have to shun people by their suffering. The next case illustrates this principle.

> A 32-year-old woman was seen in consultation because of ulcerative colitis. An array of medical regimens and surgical intervention had not changed the status of her disease. She appeared as a chronically depressed woman, obsessed by her physical condition. In psychotherapy, problems with intimacy were uncovered which accounted for past divorce and current marital difficulties. In time, the patient attempted closer interactions with other people but complained that these interpersonal relationships evoked an apprehensiveness which had previously been obscured by her stance of unhappiness.

This patient had a medical condition which improved in the course of therapy. Yet many patients with psychogenic pain or other disturbances presumed to have bases in an underlying depression are surprisingly resistant to help. The physical symptoms become an integral part of their functioning and assume a prominent place in their lifestyle, lending a certain perverse meaning to their lives. Like the delusion to which the patient clings lest he is faced with the despair of reality, patients with somatic symptoms do not easily relinquish them unless the clinician can offer something better in their place. The secondary gains and symbolic value of suffering are enormous and no simple medication will overcome these conditions. In the above case, the patient required over a year of rather intensive psychotherapy before she could give vent to her underlying sadness about a compromised marriage, something she was unwilling to admit to before. Thus, the therapy actually converted the somatic symptoms into a more overt clinical depression, a somewhat paradoxical outcome of "treatment." Indeed, many patients who become more affectively aware during the course of their psychotherapy come to realize that they have been made more sad, not less, as the physician has "taken away" the somatic symptoms which so monopolized their lives. Ultimately, the true depression can be dealt with in dynamic psychotherapy but the patient and therapist always wonder if the price to be paid for this venture is worth it. Antidepressants are not indicated.

Psychotherapy should be considered even when depressions are effectively relieved by antidepressant medication. Patients prone to depressions are often those with obsessive-compulsive characteristics who isolate emotions and have a lack of affective awareness. Individual or group therapy may help sensitize them to feelings in a way conducive to future functioning. This is very necessary, since many of these patients are overwhelmed by depressions which appear to descend upon them very mysteriously. When they can identify areas of psychodynamic vulnerability more carefully, they can anticipate precipitating factors such as specific losses or rejections and deal with them more realistically.

Some patients take to the lengthier postdepression therapeutic work willingly. For example, insight about anaclitic dependency upon others may sensitize them to this aspect of social functioning to the point where healthier object choice and relationships are possible. On the other hand, other patients may run from the confrontation with their weaknesses and wish immediate symptomatic improvement only, being intolerant of explorative work. These patients may disappear after a remission.

This recent case example illustrates, in addition, the problem of somatization seen in hysterical states and more classic psychosomatic conditions. Most clinicians are familiar with the chronically complaining patient with numerous physical ailments who defies accurate diagnosis and treatment. The aches and pains of these patients are often viewed as depressive equivalents and indicative of a patient who cannot speak of depression, but must translate it into body language. Similar formulations have been made for psychosomatic illnesses such as hypertension, asthma, or dermatologic conditions. Here, underlying conflicts leading to anger or disappointment cannot be expressed and are translated into organ dysfunction. The exacerbation of such symptoms is often loss or threatened loss, and depression plays a prominent role in both as a precipitating factor and an underlying dynamic.

Allied to the above phenomena are the so-called "masked" or "atypical" depressions (22). Here a variety of behaviors, rather than somatic conditions have been inferentially perceived as being despondencies which cannot be otherwise articulated. Children and adolescents who are not prone to describe their inner sadnesses may become enuretic, develop school phobias, become truant, demonstrate poor school performance, or become involved in antisocial acts (1).

These views of somatization, psychosomatic illness, or behaviors as variants of affective states are often simplistic for patients exhibiting such disorders often have other difficulties in the area of object relations or self-esteem. The matter is brought up because drugs are often given for these conditions. Supportive therapy is the method of choice for the hypochondriacal patient with depression who will only experience the side-effects of antidepressant medication. Many of these patients have already been unsuccessfully treated with arrays of analgesics and antianxiety drugs. Hypnosis may be useful for certain conditions of pain such as headaches.

It is problematic to view "masked" or "atypical" depressions in a conceptual framework suitable for pharmacologic treatment. The widely disparate nature of symptoms coupled with the fact that vegatative symptoms of depression such as sleep disturbance, anorexia, or psychomotor retardation are absent make the rationale for antidepressants imperfect. Generally speaking, despondencies hypothesized to exist by the clinician but not verbalized by the patient or not manifested in the form of typical symptoms respond only idiosyncratically to antidepressant medication. This is true both for adults and children. It is as though the clinician must first, in psychotherapy, elucidate a core mood disorder which the patient can appreciate and discern as a dysphoric state. Only then is consideration of antidepressant therapy possible, although it is precisely at that point that the therapist may wish to work through the central despondency psychodynamically, rather than resolving it quickly with pharmacologic agents. The next case further illustrates the process of elucidating depression.

A 33-year-old psychopath was in treatment as a condition of probation. He took a new job and was required to perform what he considered to be menial tasks, laboring long hours in order to do the work correctly. His finances were low as he had previously embarked upon a spending spree. Accordingly, he had to find a second job at night. These two ventures caused a considerable drop in self-esteem and the patient felt keenly humiliated. In time, he demonstrated despondency, apathy, and complained of insomnia and weight loss. In individual sessions, he appeared sad and depleted. Mild suicidal ideation was verbalized.

The patient was placed on imipramine medication 25 mg q.i.d. Over the span of several weeks his mood improved and he continued to function.

This case shows the development of depression in patients ordinarily considered characterologically incapable of experiencing truly despondent states. However, the diagnosis of a personality disorder does not rule out depression and patients with severely disturbed personality disorders are not immune from true affective shifts. In this case, the clinician decided to treat the patient for fear that he would abandon his job and engage in some other kind of destructive act such as leaving town or stealing funds. Ordinarily, this patient did appear to handle depression by translating it into avoidant behavior and becoming self-indulgent and fiscally irresponsible. Part of the therapy was geared toward alerting him to his depressions so that he could recognize them and reflect, rather than translate painful affect into some aberrant behavior which was ultimately detrimental for him. Patients of the type described above value their vigilance and manipulative skills; it was felt that side-effects should be kept minimal in order to encourage the medication compliance. Accordingly, a small dosage was prescribed. There was probably a significant placebo effect.

It should be again noted that until the patient was able to experience the particular dysphoric state of sadness by responding to the concomitant bodily cues and becoming affectively aware of his somatic state, antidepressants were probably of limited use. As previously mentioned, much of what is often labeled as a "masked" depression represents conjecture only and is not amenable to pharmacologic control. The patient does not see the need to take the pills since he does not experience sadness. When depression undergoes phenomenologic transformation into pain or behavior, it appears to become a different disease entity requiring alternate therapies; i.e., intensive verbal or milieu therapy.

In the previous chapter on psychoses, it was mentioned that the content of the psychotic illness could in time be discussed with the patient. However, a withholding of medication in acute psychosis is generally inhumane and contributes but a limited amount with regard to an understanding of the disease process. This is not quite as true in the affective disorders where there is a greater need to understand the nature of depression and the conditions under which it arose. Obviously, one does not allow the patient to suffer but certain patients do "seal over" quickly when antidepressant medication is administered. When this is likely to be the case, it may be prudent to withhold medication for a brief period of time in the interests of psychodynamic understanding which can occur during insight therapy. The following case illustrates this point.

A 45-year-old woman teacher was seen because of a marked depression following a sabbatical from the college where she taught. The patient had moved from another part of the country. She verbalized feelings of strangeness in a new location, and yearned to be back home. On face value, that depression was in part situational. Despite her profound sadness, she functioned relatively well and was not suicidal. Accordingly, antidepressants were withheld pending some exploratory work in treatment. Here it was learned that what had precipitated her depression was separation from an older female teacher with whom the patient had a strong affective bond. There was an unrecognized homosexual attraction. In the course of therapy, much was learned about this dynamic with a reduction in her symptoms of depression.

Medication was withheld from this patient since the clinician sensed that there was insufficient grounds for her depression. That is, the simple movement from one geographic locale to another did not seem a plausible cause for her severe despondency. While a risky venture, the delay in administering drugs confirmed the hypothesis of the clinician that there was another unspoken precipitant for her illness. Some patients do develop a depression for reasons which do not quite ring true. In these cases, given the cooperation of the patients, some exploratory work can be done in lieu of the prompt administration of medication. Other patients, probably a majority, are intolerant of such attitudes and request medication promptly. In some patients, the guilt is so strong that they request a "strong" and "severe" medication in order to suffer more; this dynamic must be noted and explored (25). The withholding of medication, as well as its administration, is a tactic which obviously colors any therapeutic relationship and the concomitant transference. Since many depressed patients feel bereft and in need of nurturance, tactics of delay may evoke anger and threaten the alliance. However, the clinician can point out to the patient his reasons for the delay and inform him that he wishes to learn a little bit more about the precipitants before the medication is begun so that a fuller improvement ensues and so that the patient does not become vulnerable to another depression in the future. Even though antidepressants take several weeks to work, the placebo value of the drug may lead to some improvement so that the patient does not reveal the dynamics of the depression. Hence, if delay is seen as clinically valid, it is wiser not to give any medication at all for a while.

Another instance of when to withhold antidepressant medication is during grief work. Some patients come to the psychiatrist profoundly depressed over a loss. Upon review, an inadequate grieving process may be detected. There are always reasons for this; the grief may be overwhelming and defended against by denial, or the patient may have underlying angers which cannot be ventilated in the normal process of grief work. Exploration of these matters is a psychotherapeutic endeavor which should not be obscured by early symptomatic relief. However, as mentioned earlier, there are some cases in which antidepressant affect may be necessary to mobilize the patient to begin grief work in the first place. Thus, the administration of antidepressant medication may facilitate psychotherapy by increasing psychomotor activity which in turn enables the patient to ventilate. In addition, the improved cognitive functioning allows the patient to more clearly see the nature of despondencies and to gaze at underlying dynamics with a greater clarity.

Therapists with a psychoanalytic orientation often perceive the administration of drugs as strongly shaping the transference. While distortions are inevitable whenever the therapist takes an active stance in the treatment, most things can be worked out with patients as long as they are analyzed (25). The risks of incurring anger by a patient who is not properly medicated outweighs the hazards of acting with conservatism in administering a drug designed to ease the burden of suffering.

The role of antidepressants in the therapy of patients prone to suicidal acts will be discussed in the context of the next case example.

A 20-year-old woman was admitted after suicidal behavior. Following financial difficulties and the loss of her boyfriend and quarrels with the father, the patient overdosed with 30 chlordiazepoxide and 40 thioridazine tablets and slit her wrists. The patient related a history of two previous suicide attempts, and related weight loss, and feelings of "depression." She had minimal psychological insight and was hostile on the ward. With 2 days of hospitalization, she stated that her suicide attempt was an attention getting device and that she no longer felt the need to die. In less than a week, she appeared more cheerful and left the hospital with tentative plans to begin individual psychotherapy. No medications were prescribed.

Patients with severe characterologic disturbances may, in moments of crisis, make serious suicidal gestures or attempts and be hospitalized, only to reconstitute rapidly within a nurturant milieu and repudiate any introspection which could avert such suicidal actions in the future. In the above case, the prognosis was bleak given the history of her multiple suicide attempts. In addition, the poor outlook was compounded by her lack of introspection which might have made the identification of psychodynamic variables available to her for future comfort. Fortunately, the clinician in this case elected not to treat her with antidepressants since he recognized that the patient, although "depressed," and showing some vegatative signs associated with despondency did not demonstrate a core mood disorder responsive to medication. In addition, she was unreliable so that administration of antidepressant medication was hazardous. Her panic states resulted in behavior culminating in suicide gestures. Emptiness, despair, and despondency were dimly perceived by her but not identified as psychological problems requiring some form of treatment. Immediate relief appeared to be afforded by hospitalization. It was doubtful whether or not the patient would continue outpatient treatment. Most likely, such treatment would be time limited only and discontinued by the patient upon discussion of painful issues; the insight or reflective process concurrent with psychotherapy would be sufficiently anxiety producing as to force the patient to seek its avoidance.

Problems with the expression of aggression also enter the picture. The above patient could not adequately give vent to her anger at her boyfriend and father. Instead, the anger became internalized, resulting in the sudden and unpremeditated overdose and angry self-mutilation. Suicide gestures and attempts often represent desires to quench extremely painful affective states of rage more than the finalization of plans to die. The point was mentioned in the previous discussion on borderline patients. With regard to depression, the clinician must recognize that many of these patients become overwhelmed by affective states of anger they cannot handle and seek an overdose of medication as a way of numbing themselves. Unfortunately, the patients are pharmacologically naive and primitive thinking enters the process so that an all or none effect ensues; the patient takes 20 pills rather than one, thinking that 20 pills will produce 20 times the effect at $\frac{1}{20}$ the speed ordinarily required. While antipsychotic agents rarely lead to death upon overdose even when massive amounts are taken, a week's supply of antidepressants can be a lethal dose due to anticholinergic poisoning and cardiovascular toxicity. Thus, it is wiser for manipulative patients prone to misuse drugs to be considered candidates for antianxiety agents as previously discussed. Drugs of the benzodiazepine class can be given more safely and do reduce panic and rage states which form such a deleterious accompaniment to the depressions.

There is occasionally hesitation on the part of clinicians to prescribe drugs which are not antidepressants for patients who have made serious suicide attempts. This reflects concern about issues of peer review as well as liability. The fear is that the patient may overdose again with the exact medication which the physician has prescribed or that colleagues may wonder why an antianxiety agent has been given to a patient who has been "depressed" and made a suicide attempt. Education is the answer to this problem. The clinician must explain his rationale for drug choice both in the patient's chart and to others. This includes addressing inevitable concerns about dependency which will be discussed in the next chapter. For the moment, it is sufficient to recognize that it may be better for a high risk patient to rely upon a benzodiazepine than to engage in repetitive suicide attempts which, statistically speaking, may well culminate in a lethal act.

Concern is also often expressed to the effect that patients who really want to commit suicide will "do it anyway" and limitations on drug prescriptions will not deter them as they can always purchase additional medications. Yet it should be recalled that it is not the number of pills prescribed that determine behavior, but the verbal message which accompanies the prescription. Limited dosages given with some discussion of the clinician's concern for safety and the fact that he is giving the patient only a small quantity of pills conveys a concern. The patient, additionally, can be counselled to call the doctor if he feels more despondent or if he needs to be seen sooner.

As patients improve or are placed on maintenance medication, some leniency on prescriptions is possible. For some patients on divided dose regimens of antidepressants, or lithium, one week's supply imposes an inconvenience and can result in significantly higher costs since pharmacist's costs are reduced with larger unit quantities such as 100. These factors must be borne in mind.

An incomplete suicidal act or gesture often provides some relief for the patient. Unless the behavior was the culmination of a well thought out plan for death or represented delusional thinking or hallucinatory activity, the act itself serves a bizarre catharsis which makes the patient unwilling to engage in further therapeutic work. The clinician might logically expect that a patient who had taken an overdose or cut her wrists might view the pathologic nature of this activity, question its origins, and seek help. Regrettably, this is not the case and the attention seeking component, as verbalized by the patient in the above case example, is extremely successful and has great mobilizing value. Yet while the patient himself may seek little help, relatives and friends are often adamant in their demands upon the therapist that "something be done," including the use of medication, to avoid further catastrophe. In such instances, the therapist must stand firm and point out to parents that it is the patient who must experience dysphoria and that medication is only useful for those who are responsive to such despondency and utilize it in the service of alleviating depressed mood. Whether or not the clinician then gives the patient medication to gratify some nurturant need with the hope of enticing the latter in therapy is dependent upon the situation.

The use of drugs following resolution of acute depression will be exemplified by the next example.

> A 50-year-old man complained of loss of energy. The patient related insomnia, with early morning awakening, impotence, and general fatigue with anorexia and weight loss. These symptoms followed an industrial accident leading to the loss of a digit of one hand.
>
> He was placed on amitriptyline 150 mg per day with improvement of his symptoms.
>
> In time, on an outpatient basis, the dose was reduced to 50 mg over a 7-month period, but the patient complained of a recurrence of his depression. Hence the dose was elevated to 100 mg with alleviation of mood disturbance. A second reduction in dose to 50 mg h.s. was attempted about 1½ years after the initial depression. The patient appeared comfortable on that regimen.

This case illustrates problems of maintenance dosage. Maintenance antidepressant medication is generally perceived as being necessary for approximately 3 to 6 months following remission from an acute depressive illness. The reasons for this time interval relates to the cyclical aspect of depression which can have a time span of 6 months or longer; patients treated during the early stages of depression may show a remission only to relapse before the cycle is complete. Remissions which occur in the structure of the hospital may also represent a "flight into health." Upon discharge, lack of structure and support and sharp confrontation with reality may lead to relapse. Once the time interval of 6 months has elapsed, the patient's dose of antidepressants can be gradually tapered over a several week interval so that the clinician can monitor recurrence of depressive symptoms. Tapering also prevents the cholinergic effects which might come with abrupt cessation. Maintenance dosage is usually ½ that required during the acute phase of depression. In time, further reduction may be attempted as tolerated. The clinician should always consider abstinence periods for patients on maintenance antidepressant medication. When drug withdrawals are attempted depends upon the periodicity of the depressive bouts and their intensity and frequency. Timing is also important; if the patient typically becomes depressed at a specific time of year, antidepressants should not be withdrawn at that time. If the patient is under or anticipates significant life stress, drugs should not be discontinued. Otherwise, a trial period without medication may allow the therapist to view functioning and determine the necessity for pharmacologic therapy. In the above case, drugs were withdrawn after 7 months but appeared still to be needed. The patient remained on antidepressants continuously for over 1½ years, a relatively long time. Some patients require such extended treatments but the majority of depressed patients do not; thus, there is an absence of long-term toxicities as described in the literature.

Risk of relapse is always a concern of patients. However, relapse is not explosive. Furthermore, psychotherapy may bring about changes in coping mechanisms which decrease the patient's susceptibility to depression. Patients develop insight into incipient depression and medication can be started promptly.

Some patients prone to recurrent depressive episodes may be responsive to an altogether different pharmacologic agent, lithium. Such responsiveness represents the existence of a different psychopathological process which will now be discussed.

> A 32-year-old woman suffered a moderately severe depression upon moving to another city. An occupant of a large house without any neighbors close by, she felt increasingly lonely and isolated; in addition, her husband took a job which required that he kept longer hours. She was treated with antidepressants and psychotherapy. A remission occurred but a second depression followed within 6 months preceded by a mild hypomanic state. At this point, another review was made of her history with the finding that she was prone to mild mood swings and that her mother had experienced profound alterations of mood as long as the patient could recall. The patient was then begun on lithium carbonate and maintained on the drug without recurrence of an affective disorder over the ensuing 4 years.

This case illustrates the possible utility of lithium in the treatment of affective disease. In the above case, the disease had some of the clinical characteristics of a bipolar illness characterized by hypomania and depression, a condition for which lithium is less indicated than a "purer" bipolar illness with periods of distinct mania interspersed with depression.

The fact that a recurrent affective illness such as depression might warrant a simple salt rather than a more complex psychopharmacologic agent such as an antidepressant makes it an affective disorder nosologically quite different. There are also phenomenologic differences which lie in the cyclical nature of the depression or manic attacks. Thus, one depression justifies antidepressant therapy with possible maintenance; two depressions may also justify a similar regimen, but two or more may also raise the possibility of the illness being an undetected unipolar or bipolar disease warranting consideration of lithium. The relative potency of lithium in stabilizing mood has led to its use when even a first depressive illness occurs; currently, some clinicians treat a solitary depression with antidepressants and subsequently with maintenance lithium if they discover that the patient has been depressed before, or hypomanic, or has a history of recurrent mood swings, or a family history suggestive of a unipolar or bipolar affective disease. Whether or not such treatment is efficacious depends upon the individual case. In the above instance, the patient was treated with maintenance antidepressants for approximately 6 months after which time drugs were stopped. The recurrence of a second depression preceded by hypomanic episode led the clinician to wonder whether the patient might have a bipolar illness manifested by recurrent depressive bouts with interspersed hypomania. Lithium was tried partly on empirical grounds, given some historical data mildly supportive of a cyclical illness. The existence of a strong family history of manic-depressive illness would have strengthened the indication for lithium. Had the patient only experienced recurrent depressions, lithium might have been helpful although the literature is still inconclusive in this regard (15).

It should be noted that lithium in the above case was used as a prophylactic agent and not as an antidepressant. The properties of lithium as an antidepressant are still not fully established. The drug acts to prevent the occurrence of depression in bipolar disease; if started only during a depression, there may be no effect or possibly some attenuation of the depression. Yet even when lithium is prescribed for well documented bipolar disease when the patient is stable, depression may occur and reflect the need for dose adjustment. In some instances, concurrent use of antidepressants is necessary. Lithium appears to protect against the activation of a hypomanic or manic state by antidepressants.

The above patient was placed on the maintenance dose of 900 mg in three daily divided dosages. Her serum levels on this regimen were 0.7 mEq/L. Adequate maintenance serum levels vary, depending upon patient. Serum levels of 0.6 to 1.2 have been mentioned as desirable by manufacturers of the drug. Dosages leading to levels of 1.0 to 1.5 are generally reserved for acute manic episodes while serum levels between 1.5 to 2.0 can be associated with toxicity. Thus, lithium, unlike antipsychotic and antidepressant drugs, is a psychopharmacologic agent which can be monitored readily through serum determinations since it is not protein bound and is not metabolized in the body.

Lithium is the drug of choice for mania; yet several days are required until antimanic effects appear due to body equilibration. Consequently, supplemental antipsychotic medications are useful in the initial stages of treatment. The following case example illustrates this principle.

A 49-year-old male was hospitalized because of grandiosity, hyperactivity, and delusions. The patient was attempting to write novels, bought a piano he did not know how to play, and stopped going to work. He impulsively married and lavishly bought gifts. He was eventually brought to the hospital by his relatives where he presented a manic picture with agitation and hyperactivity. Lithium carbonate was begun in a dose of

1500 mg per day and eventually increased to 1800 mg per day. However, the agitation persisted and thioridazine 100 mg per day was added to this regimen. After several weeks, the patient showed a decrease in his manic activity and the thioridazine was eventually discontinued.

In the above instance, thioridazine was used to control the patient until lithium exerted its effect. Any antipsychotic agent is efficacious although manic patients often prefer non-sedating antipsychotic agents and struggle against effects caused by drugs which make them feel lethargic. Generally, the clinician should wait 5 to 7 days until the serum level is in the therapeutic range for mania. Then, the antipsychotic can be slowly tapered to ascertain whether or not the patient's mood is normalized by the lithium. In the event that agitation reappears with the reduction of the antipsychotic agent, the latter can be restored and lithium can be titrated higher and adjusted to an appropriate serum level.

Lithium affects the psychotic behavior associated with mania, but by itself possesses no antipsychotic properties. Rather, it appears to induce a remission in the thought disorder of manic-depressive psychoses by normalizing mood. In this regard, lithium is similar to antidepressants in treating certain psychotic depressions.

A relatively wide dose range may be required to induce therapeutic blood levels in the manic state. A starting t.i.d. or q.i.d. regimen is common and upward titration may be carried out over a few days as was the case in the above example. Blood samples may be obtained every 3 or 4 days in the acute phase to ascertain whether the therapeutic levels are being reached.

Serum sampling must be made 12 hours after ingestion of the last dose. Lithium is absorbed after 6 to 8 hours, so that 12 hours allows for equilibration. Patients need to be told that having blood drawn earlier may result in spuriously higher "peak" values which are inaccurate. They must also be instructed to take their previous dose, since lower values will occur otherwise. Education is vital in this matter since patients quite naturally assume that the blood levels are constant and do not vary.

Serum sampling is one facet of manic-depressive illness which distinguishes it from other psychiatric disorders and imparts to the disease and treatment a more "medical" flavor. This is both good and bad. Analogies made between lithium and replacement hormones such as insulin may foster compliance, and the patient may feel less stigmatized by the perception that his illness is "biochemical." On the other hand, the disorder is not just a one of mood but a psychiatric illness with many other parameters of dysfunction including object relations. Many patients are narcissistic in character structure and sensitive to losses which in the past have triggered mood swings. These issues deserve exploration in psychotherapy.

The fact that the clinician must monitor serum levels makes him particularly cognizant to the exact dose, a sometimes alarming venture which sensitizes him to a precision he is not used to when it comes to psychopharmacology. Antipsychotic and antidepressant agents are generally given with wide margins of safety and with wide latitudes with regard to dose. In contrast, the toxicity of lithium is greatly feared because it is associated with such a discrete end point. Familiarity with lithium will increase the comfort of the clinician.

On the other hand, the availability of a serum value to monitor "progress" can make the clinician complacent and less apt to see the patient in the office, where finer examination of mood is best carried out. Some clinicians order a serum lithium level every month, a costly endeavor that sheds little or no light on the clinical functioning of the patient. Frequent levels are useful in early stages of acute control or maintenance. Thereafter, serum determinations are indicated on the basis of clinical findings or changes in physical health.

While serum levels of lithium may normally fluctuate as much as 100% during the day (30), the intake of lithium by the patient is not as critical as it might seem or analogous to, say, anti-coagulants. Generally, missed doses can be made up if the patient is tolerant of the possible nausea which results from a double dose. Some patients tolerate 600 mg of the drug at once, thus facilitating dose consolidation. Generally, dosages above this lead to transient toxicities. The main requirement for lithium appears to be that it is taken regularly and that the patient receives his required daily dosage. Nevertheless, for some patients in early recovery, dosages of 1200 or 1500 mg will mean t.i.d. or even q.i.d. regimens, necessitating some attention to the pill taking process. Some patients have not thought about the purchase of a pill box. Reminders to take medications are necessary. Some patients in homes without children put the bottle of lithium on the breakfast table to remind themselves while others retain the bottle near a central place, next to car keys or wallet or carry additional supplies in a briefcase.

Some patients with rather classic bipolar affective disease cannot be treated with lithium because they are too unreliable. There is a need for compliance on the part of the patient, particularly since the drug is a prophylactic agent and may be discontinued when the patient feels normal. Seriously depressed patients who are suicidal or those who will not adhere to the necessary treatment regimen may be poor candidates for the drug even though the medication appears clinically indicated. In fact, lithium has a usefulness occasionally dictated more by the relative psychological integrity of the patient than by the illness which gives rise to its consideration in the first place. This is particularly true as the drug finds use in an array of conditions where mood swings are seen, including certain schizophrenic illness or personality disorders.

Patients generally ask how long they may be on lithium since they have heard that some patients require the drug for several years. Evidence is slowly emerging that lithium, like all drugs, is not free of long-term toxicities. Renal lesions have been reported in some patients with lithium-induced nephrogenic diabetes insipidis (2). Thyroid dysfunction may also occur. Thus, like all drugs, indefinite maintenance is not justified without consideration of risk. Maintenance therapy is a complex matter and, like psychosis and depressions, depends upon the severity and frequency of the attack (27). Each case must be individualized. One manic attack may not necessarily justify long-term maintenance although catastrophic manic episodes which come about suddenly and lead the patient to deplete family finances may influence the issue of maintenance lithium. Requirements for lithium appear to decrease with age, a fact generally applicable to all drugs. In addition, manic-depressive illness may decrease in severity with advancing years. When spans between mood swings lengthen, abstinence can be considered. Patients who experience, say, one mild manic or depressive episode a year may be candidates for lithium-free periods, particularly if they have good therapeutic rapport with the clinician and can, with the aid of family, notify him at the onset of a severe mood change. While hypomania is not willingly acknowledged as illness by many patients, some can sense when they are "getting high;" lithium at that time can be instituted and continued for several months. Anticipated major psychological stress may warrant reinstitution of the drug also.

It is important that any patient being withdrawn from lithium be closely monitored by the clinician, not just for the sake of detecting the onset of mania or depression, but to assess finer cognitive functioning as well. Lithium may induce complex behavioral alterations beyond the simple stabilization of mood. Patients may talk about changes in levels of irritability or frustration tolerance or describe subtle changes in their ability to take criticism at work or even perform tasks requiring concentration. Levels of fatigability may change. These fine parameters of functioning, when balanced against toxicities, may help shape a decision to resume or not resume lithium prophylaxis.

Lithium does not make a patient immune from affect. Patients on lithium may still get despondent and can "feel things," a concern they often verbalize before the onset of treatment. Affective awareness is retained but curbs appear to be placed on the extent to which patients oscillate with regard to mood. For certain people who show heightened productivity during states of mild euphoria or hypomania, the use of lithium may be problematic although little data exist in this regard. What is often verbalized by patients who have been manic at one point in their illness is the desire to again experience the "high" during which they became euphoric, grandiose, and expansive. The endogenous "high" is not unlike the activation obtained from central nervous system stimulants use in that there is a sense of power and well being; thus, the "high" is a positive affective state even though the patient well recognizes that catastrophic results can occur from false joviality which leads him to make errors in judgment with regard to finances, job, or family. Patients on lithium may experiment with it in order to induce the "high" and some watchfulness has to be maintained in certain types of patients who, while wishing help, also mourn the absence of euphoria which they once had. Such a loss must be acknowledged with the patient and becomes an issue in psychotherapy.

The skill of handling lithium is dependent upon knowledge of its toxicities. The salt is excreted by the kidneys, and adequate renal function dictates its use and safety. Baseline renal tests are required. Changes in urinary function must be reported by the patient. The patient should also inform the physician if he develops cardiovascular disease which involves prescriptions for diuretics or a low salt diet, both of which may lead to the lowered serum sodium and potentially increased lithium. As an electrolyte, lithium also may induce cardiac irregularities. Hence, baseline EKGs in elderly patients or those at risk for cardiovascular disease are prudent.

The symptoms of lithium intoxication follow the expected toxicities of any electrolyte imbalance and include central nervous system dysfunction which progresses from fine tremor to disorientation and coma. Toxicities can be monitored clinically, and confirmed with serum level tests although in rare instances a normal serum level may exist in the face of toxicity.

Patients do not often think about matters pertaining to fluid intake and output and require some education in this area. Excessive concern on the part of the physician and patient about sodium loss often attends the use of lithium during hot weather when sweating occurs. In a healthy person, homeostatic mechanisms generally regulàte body electrolytes and supplemental salt is not needed. Excessive thirst and urinary frequency may be symptoms of a polyuria-polydipsia syndrome which is not uncommon in patients and presumed to result from antidiuretic hormone changes induced by the drug. The condition is usually benign but it must be monitored; it may influence the continued use of lithium since, as previously mentioned, alterations may not always be reversible.

Lithium has the unexpected potential to induce hypothyroidism. Therefore, baseline thyroid studies are desirable before the onset of therapy. Altered thyroid function may represent long-term toxicity. Again such a development should make the clinician reflect on the risk/benefit ratio of continued lithium use.

Within the last several years, the anticonvulsant carbamazepine (Tegretol) has been used as an alternative to lithium for cases in which the patient is refractory to the latter salt (26). The basis for carbamazepine's efficacy remains unclear but is thought to be due to some effect upon limbic system "kindling," a state of subcortical arousal culiminating in seizure-like affective or psychotic states. Like lithium, carbamazepine can be assayed with blood levels. The principal toxicity of the drug is the rare development of bone marrow suppression, necessitating careful clinical monitoring of the patient and periodic blood tests. Lithium and carbamazepine have been used together in the treatment of some patients whose mood swings are uncontrolled by either drug alone.

Mania is regarded as an affective disorder. From the standpoint of target symptoms, it lies on a continuum of psychomotor activation. At one end of that continuum is severe motor retardation seen in depressed states or even in psychotic conditions such as catatonia. At the other end is the hyperactive and manic patient. Agitated depressions fall near the midpoint of the continuum, as does insomnia, a condition of restlessness accompanying both depression and anxiety. Insomnia, then, is an entity which bridges the gap between discussions of depression and anxiety.

Insomnia is a symptom often associated with depression and is often the earliest signs of an impending depressive episode. Patients may complain of difficulties falling asleep or remaining asleep. Some patients may complain of sleeping too much during the daytime and being unable to sleep at night. Other patients complain of early morning awakening.

Insomnia is also one of the first symptoms to remit in patients who respond to antidepressants. However, the condition is most distressing to patients who must wait for the therapeutic effect of a drug and clinicians often prescribe hypnotic agents to induce sleep in the interim. In some instances, such a regimen is justified on a limited basis. Sleep deprivation heightens the irritability of all individuals. Night is a time of loneliness. There are few people to talk to, streets are empty, and vulnerability to personal safety is high. These anxieties, together with the recall of even more unpleasant anamnestic material derived by the patient's painful ruminations over past events contributes to his feeling worse in the morning. Even when sleep is artificially induced, it is often fitful and leaves him without the feeling of refreshment.

It is useful for the clinician to review with the patient the role sleep has played in his life. For many patients, sleep is a necessary evil while other patients enjoy sleeping and still others sleep under stress. Attention to the baseline state dictates how vigorously the clinician will wish to use pharmacologic agents. For patients who generally sleep poorly, restoration of sleep to baseline function is difficult. These patients may be quite resistant to hypnotics and simply become drowsy or feel drugged from them without experiencing the induction of true sleep. Control is often an issue in the sleep process. Paranoid patients or those individuals who are hypervigilant and anxious may see sleep as a time when they are defenseless and unable to cope with events around them. More can be done for their well being in the form of scheduled nighttime activities than the repetitious and perfunctory dispensing of drugs 1 hour before "sleep time."

Some reeducation with regard to sleep and insomnia is helpful in general. Nighttime diversion, a mundane issue, can be profitably discussed with individuals and tasks can be chosen which do not require too much concentration but put the patient in a position of "doing something." The assembly of puzzles, small kits, or models gives individuals a task oriented mission which has a definitive end point. Such measures may be preferable to the passive pursuit of watching television which is unrewarding for many individuals who relish activity and the feeling of assertion. Sleep medications can be given near midnight when the initial tension of the evening begins to wane and there exists some genuine fatigue induced by the mild activity.

Early morning awakening should be followed by the patient's rising from bed to occupy himself in some manner mentioned above. Although it may be dark and cold, particularly in the winter, patients do not generally fall asleep again and toss and turn; the bed becomes a place of torment rather than warmth or security. Hypnotics taken past 3 or 4 a.m. generally produce early morning sedation which interferes with other functions. Elderly patients who complain that they sleep very little may need reassurance from physicians to the effect that this is normal and that requirements decrease with increasing age. Companionship is often important in elderly patients and telephone discussion with another person before bedtime may be of psychological relief.

Nocturnal dosages of antidepressants do facilitate sleep through their sedative action. The barbiturates have been used for decades to induce sleep but more recently have fallen in disfavor because of their potential for abuse. The same is true of other hypnotic agents such as chloral hydrate, glutethimide (Doriden), methyprylon (Noludar), or methaqualone (Quaalude, Parest). All of these hypnotic agents can suppress rapid eye movement (REM) sleep. Some of these drugs have street value; this, together with the fact that all of the above drugs are scheduled substances, has led to their relative abandonment in clinical practice. Sleep studies comparing some of the above drugs with the benzodiazepine flurazepam (Dalmane) has shown the latter agent to be effective in inducing sleep for periods of several weeks without the development of tolerance (16, 17). Flurazepam is currently marketed rather exclusively as a hypnotic, although all longer acting benzodiazepines are potentially useful for inducing sleep by virtue of their sedative effects; none are specific for sleep as such.

The benzodiazepines can suppress REM sleep in a dose-dependent manner. However, in usual therapeutic doses, there is minimal suppression of REM sleep and no REM rebound. Use of high dosages of benzodiazepines becomes analogous to the use of barbiturates in terms of central nervous system depression, sedation, and interference with

REM sleep. High dosages of long-acting benzodiazepines including flurazepam for sleep may also lead to excessive lethargy in the elderly (8). For older patients, shorter-acting benzodiazepines such as oxazepam (Serax) may be preferred. There are several shorter acting benzodiazepines now marketed for sleep. These include temazepam (Restoril) and triazolam (Halcion).

The antianxiety agents will now be discussed. Description is limited to the benzodiazepines for reasons mentioned below. The term "minor tranquilizer," is often used to describe antianxiety compounds. It is inaccurate for several reasons. Anxiety can be phenomenologically as crippling an illness as a psychosis and is thus not minor. Tranquilizers have antipsychotic properties while antianxiety drugs do not.

Anxiety may be associated with many psychopathologic states such as psychosis and depression. Yet it complicates a regimen to add an antianxiety agent to an antipsychotic or antidepressant drug. Rather, the antipsychotic or antidepressant with the most sedative properties should be chosen to combine effects in one pharmacologic regimen.

In the discussions of affective disorders mentioned to date, it was pointed out that drugs utilized are rather specific for the restoration of mood. Antidepressants return deranged mood to normal while having no effect on patients without mood disturbances. Likewise, lithium is a normalizer of mood without any effect on normal patients. With anxiety, the situation is different. Most anxiety drugs have the potential for inducing psychological dependency since relief from anxiety is intimately bound up with pleasurable sensations. This phenomenon is seen in alcoholism, where disinhibition is a desired end point; antianxiety agents can also produce mild disinhibition at increased dosages. Hence the clinician treating patients with anxieties is immediately subject to theoretical concerns about the addictive capabilities of this class of drugs. This is reflected by the need of a narcotics classification for existing antianxiety compounds, including those of the benzodiazepine class.

In actuality, concerns about dependency and addiction appear to be overemphasized. Some work with chlordiazepoxide indicates that withdrawal occurs when amounts up to 300 mg daily are used for 1 month (13) while other clinicians have stated that dosages 10 times those of therapeutic ranges are required to produce dependency (31). The vast majority of patients do not escalate their intake to these levels. There are a few isolated case reports in which patients receiving conservative dosages of benzodiazepines for long periods of time have developed withdrawal reactions, including seizures and psychosis, when such drugs have been abruptly withdrawn. Considering the vastness of benzodiazepine usage, however, such reports appear quite infrequent; workers in the field of drug abuse have commented on the relative safety of benzodiazepine administration. Many of these drugs have comparatively long half lives and active metabolites so that blood levels become gradually reduced upon cessation of the drugs (9).

Yet concern about the abuse of antianxiety drugs continues, largely in the absence of data and based more upon moralistic concerns. The benzodiazepines continue to be among the most widely prescribed drugs in the United States. A complication of the popularity of these drugs is patient demand. Patients come to expect these drugs and physicians in practice will find the situation analogous to penicillin; if they do not prescribe either of the two, their clientele may go elsewhere looking for the appropriate medication. Thus, at the outset, the clinician is faced with a burden that he does not see to the same extent with antidepressants or antipsychotic agents.

Another more formidable burden is posed by the need to differentiate pathologic from nonpathologic conditions. Anxiety is a ubiquitous human emotion; it is a component of all illness and is associated with all forms of social stress. Hence, antianxiety compounds can be easily viewed as necessary drugs for all medical conditions and situational reactions. Most anxiety remits with supportive care. Of all conditions in psychiatry, anxiety is the most ill-defined and shows the greatest response to nonspecific factors (28). For example, studies have shown that chronically anxious patients do well on drugs but do poorly on placebo whereas patients who have only experienced anxiety for a short time do exceedingly well on both. Lower class patients often expect the treatment of anxiety to involve sedation in order that they "feel something" while upper class patients wish an antianxiety agent which is precisely devoid of sedation and in no way interferes with daily functioning.

As nonspecific as are the factors influencing antianxiety drug response, so are the target symptoms and syndromes identified as responsive to these agents. Internists and family practitioners see a host of illnesses with such associated complaints and prescribe antianxiety agents with benefit. For the psychiatric patient, an attempt must be made to differentiate, qualitatively and quantitatively, the nature of the anxiety. There is a wide difference between the anxiety resulting from an anticipated airplane ride and the panic state felt by the patient who fears the loss of control and the breakthrough of a psychosis; some anxieties, as described previously, represent heightened vigilance leading to paranoia. Other anxieties are seen in borderline syndromes and reflect primary process ideation. Many patients are chronically anxious individuals as illustrated in the following example.

> A 53-year-old woman was seen in the clinic because of "nerves." The patient herself had a history of hypertension which required a rather strict diet and medication. Her general personality was hysterical in nature, manifested by flamboyant gestures, dress, and speech. She appeared quite labile and over-demonstrative in describing her many life difficulties. She had gone to many physicians and had been prescribed a vast array of medications, ranging from barbiturates to antipsychotic drugs. None of these provided any relief until she was placed on diazepam (Valium) 30 mg q.d.

This case illustrates several principles in the management of anxiety. First, it should be evident to the clinician that there is an array of terms used to describe the condition of anxiety. Expressions such as "nerves," "tension," and other somatic phrases may describe the general state of anxiety which is either attached to a particular behavior or event or may be more "free floating." Literature regarding antianxiety agents has usually stressed their use in "free floating" anxiety and panic-like states; there is the implication that these conditions reflect "truer" and more valid affective disorders as opposed to a situational or environmentally produced stress. This implication is not borne out in clinical practice. Many patients demonstrate anxiety about clearly defined circumstances as well as anxiety which is ill-defined. The above patient had numerous good concerns for being anxious, including the deteriorating condition of a diabetic husband. Other of her anxieties had no obvious basis and their etiologies could not be elicited even in prolonged interviews. The clinician who ultimately treated her elected to use antianxiety drugs, hoping to avoid her chronic use of barbiturates or antipsychotic agents which could have more deleterious long-term effect. Thus, in a sense, the antianxiety medication was used as a substitute for another drug. In addition, it was felt that her hypertension might be helped by antianxiety medication.

It has been advocated that antianxiety agents should be only used for short periods of time (71). This statement is made partly on philosophical grounds and represents the thought that patients should learn to adapt to stress-producing situations as a matter of personal growth; the sentiment has puritanical overtones. Additionally, the statement is made because of concerns about dependency. In reality, the clinician usually finds that patients warrant antianxiety drugs for longer periods of time than a few days. In practice, patients with marked characterologic disturbances manifested by lability of mood and affect or impulsivity may require some degree of maintenance antianxiety medication to curb a general level of irritability which hampers their functioning. Some of these patients may be unreliable and require a good deal of monitoring; others, as described above, may be more tractable when closely followed. Conservative amounts of, say, diazepam or chlordiazepoxide are particularly useful for these individuals who magnify and become victims of the pressures of everyday life. Psychotherapy must accompany such drug prescriptions.

Another example of the above principle follows.

> A 30-year-old man was seen because of tension and interpersonal difficulties. He was an extremely obsessive-compulsive individual with rigid standard for excellence. He extolled perfectionistic virtues at work as well as demanding obedience from his family. All in contact with him found him extremely difficult to live with since his demeanor was such that deviations from his high expectations led to outbursts of anger and criticism. In the course of intensive psychotherapy, he was given diazepam 5 to 10 mg q.i.d. p.r.n. He eventually trusted himself to use this medication and felt calmer; this calmness then extended to those around him.

This case illustrates the use of maintenance antianxiety medication for a characterologically related tension. The anxiety was not circumscribed but pervaded many areas of the patient's life. Therapy enabled him to tolerate the drug with benefit. It is difficult to say how long such a patient should remain on medication but likely that the drug would be discontinued in time when coping mechanisms were enhanced through treatment. Actually, the patient's total weekly dose of medication was minimal and he periodically attempted his own "drug holidays." The use of p.r.n. dose schedules will be discussed shortly.

Antianxiety agents such as diazepam have been found useful in the treatment of certain agitated depressions and some work has shown this benzodiazepine to be as effective as acetophenazine (Tindal) (14). In clinical practice, the clinician is apt to see obsessional patients who become anxious and despondent when they feel they are losing control or are overwhelmed by environmental circumstances. Patients with work standards as in the above example are highly vulnerable to criticism, suffering small depressive bouts with anxiety and ruminative preoccupations. The benzodiazepines may well be the agents of choice for such target symptoms. To this extent, it may be wiser to conceptualize the dysphoric state of these patients as agitated despondencies rather than true clinical depressions.

The treatment of anxiety is always an imperfect one. A good antianxiety agent should reduce anxiety without producing lethargy. Traditionally, the barbiturates have been used in the treatment of anxiety but they are sedative drugs, producing drowsiness. Meprobamate (Miltown, Equanil) was marketed as an antianxiety agent but also produces sedation; its potential fatality with overdose and its abuse potential have cast it in disfavor. It is no more efficacious than the benzodiazepines. Of the currently marketed antianxiety agents, those offering the most rational pharmacologic utilization are the benzodiazepines. Unlike the varied classes of antipsychotic or antidepressant drugs, patient response to differing benzodiazepines is essentially the same and all benzodiazepines are roughly comparable in efficacy. Their variance relates to the biologic half-lives and presence of active metabolites. Considerations of treatment are based mainly on this fact.

Chlordiazepoxide and diazepam have half-lives from 1 to 2 days and have active metabolites. Chronic dosing with these drugs leads to steady-state levels within a week and allows the clinician to utilize infrequent daily dosing. Regimens of b.i.d. dosing may suffice. Frequently the total dose can be given at night with residual antianxiety effect during the day. Newer drugs such as prazapam (Verstran) and clorazepate (Azene, Tranxene) either have long half-lives or active metabolites with long half-lives; thus, they offer no advantage in use. Two benzodiazepines, namely oxazepam (Serax) and lorazepam (Ativan) have half-lives of hours rather than days. Both have no active metabolites and are thus particularly useful for elderly patients or those with impaired hepatic or renal function since drug accumulation is less likely to occur.

Diazepam has muscle relaxant properties and may be useful in states of anxiety associated specifically with muscle tension.

Alprazolam (Xanax) is the latest of the benzodiazepines to be marketed. As previously mentioned, it is a short acting drug which has some specific antidepressant properties which make it useful for agitated and depressive states of a mild nature.

Unlike other drugs in psychiatry such as the antipsychotic and antidepressant agents, antianxiety drugs are usually given at optimal dose from the outset. Slight adjustments upward may be needed at times and downward titration is occasionally necessary to avoid sedation. Older patients require lower doses and cumulative toxicity must be monitored.

The next example deals with dose scheduling as well as the limitation of antianxiety drug use.

> A 35-year-old man was referred because of panic states in association with business trips. The patient also suffered bouts of anxiety when giving public speeches. Analytically oriented psychotherapy produced some insight into the dynamics of his fears. However, residual anxiety persisted in the face of this insight necessitating the administration of diazepam 10 mg q.i.d. p.r.n. On this regimen, the patient showed some diminution of his anxiety associated with public appearances. However, he continued to experience tension whenever the occasion arose to travel. Yet he appeared to obtain as much solace by simply carrying the medication with him than by taking it on a regular basis.

This case illustrates both irrational and rational forms of anxiety. The irrational anxiety, perceived by the patient as an inner tremulousness and fear, occurred whenever he had to go out of town and leave home. This fear included a dread of airplanes and occurred when he had to drive an automobile long distances as well. The anxiety had phobic qualities to it. The more rational anxieties were those associated with public speaking, an apprehensiveness which even the most practiced actors and lecturers have. Theoretically, the irrational anxiety would be the target symptom most amenable to antianxiety drug control since it is more pathogenic than the symptoms associated with the normative stress of public speaking. However, many such phobic anxieties appear notoriously resistant to pharmacologic regimens.

Deconditioning paradigms have shown some promise. The antidepressant imipramine has been described as aborting the actual panic attack though leaving untouched the anticipatory anxiety which still requires therapy (18). This form of treatment is still experimental and the mechanisms of action of the drug are unexplained. The matter will be discussed further in relation to the use of the same agent in the therapy of enuresis and school phobia.

In the above case, diazepam was given to the patient on a p.r.n. regimen basis. While it has been stated previously that nocturnal dosing may be sufficient, this patient needed to keep tight control on his own drugs and was fearful of "becoming addicted." To this extent, he was urged to manage his own medication and take dosages as needed. Many patients with anxiety wish relief from this disabling symptom, yet are as anxious about the medication they take as they are uncomfortable with their own affective disorder. Certain obsessive-compulsive individuals who place a premium on independence dislike antianxiety medication although they appreciate the fact that it alleviates some of their chronic level of tension. If they can take the medication on their own schedule, they feel more in control. Merely owning the drug has psychological significance and allows the patient to feel that he can master the environment.

On the other hand, some patients with the need for conformity and adherence to schedules do poorly with a p.r.n. regimen and feel better when precise schedules of drug intake are advised. Thus, these patients are told to take a conservative dose of the same drug exactly 6 hours apart during the day to alleviate stress. The ritual in itself may alleviate anxiety. It is often difficult to anticipate which patient will do better on a fixed schedule and which patient will prefer a p.r.n. regimen. Generally, the patient will settle the issue when asked; thus, questions about work habits and matters of daily routine will establish the level of perfectionism inherent in the patient's personality. Some patients will quite freely talk about preferring to take a medication only "when needed." For others, the behavior of drug intake will determine the matter for if the patient is prescribed a fixed dose, he may return for follow-up and inform the clinician that he has changed to a p.r.n. schedule.

Schedules of p.r.n. medication are contraindicated for individuals prone to misuse antianxiety drugs. Patients with addictive traits must be dispensed measured amounts of drugs. Estimates of usage by the therapist are mandatory. This tactic of questioning whether a new prescription is warranted on the basis of the number of pills previously dispensed will cast the therapist in a new light of being an enforcer or policeman. There is no way of changing this except to handle it openly and make trust the therapeutic issue.

The benzodiazepines are remarkably safe and no deaths have been reported from overdose unless such abuse has been associated with the ingestion of other drugs or alcohol. Yet it is still imprudent to prescribe amounts over 100 or numerous refills of smaller amounts. It is preferable, instead, to prescribe a week's supply and have the patient return or at least keep in telephone contact in order to ascertain future drug needs.

Side-effects of the benzodiazepines when used in the treatment of anxiety are excessive central nervous system depression. Otherwise, side-effects are rare and do not constitute significant contraindications to use. It is noteworthy that unlike other sedatives used for the treatment of anxieties such as the barbiturates, the benzodiazepines cause no liver microsomal enzyme induction. Hence, no major drug interactions have been observed outside of cumulative central nervous system depressant effects from the combination of these drugs with alcohol.

One rare adverse reaction of particular note has been reported with these drugs. Disinhibitory phenomenon leading to "paradoxical" rage responses or suicidal ideation have been reported with all of the benzodiazepines except oxazepam. To some extent, these reactions may be more a function of drug effects in certain patient populations than true toxicities. Thus, obsessional or paranoid patients may react to exogenously induced relaxation or sedation by becoming more excited, not less. This disinhibitory phenomenon has in part been discussed in the treatment of borderline and paranoid conditions where benzodiazepines have been recommended as a means of acceptably reducing hypervigilance in patients who cannot tolerate the more severe side-effects of antipsychotic medication. "Paradoxical" responses are basically disinhibitory in nature. Pharmacologic disinhibition is more ubiquitous than realized, occurring most commonly with the ingestion of alcohol. For large groups of patients, alcohol produces many untoward psychological effects including the release of anger and rage. Although alcohol is initially taken to relax, excess leads to cortical disinhibition and results in exaggeration of certain premorbid depressive or antisocial traits in individuals so predisposed. As for antianxiety drugs, there is no evidence that giving benzodiazepines to patients prone to aggression or poor impulse control leads to exacerbation of these propensities (23).

The reasons for the absence of the implication of oxazepam in paradoxical rage reactions is unclear but may well relate to the fact that this drug is metabolized so quickly and does not accumulate within the body. While it is not known which types of individuals are susceptible to "paradoxical" reactions, it appears reasonable to view patients with characterologic structure of severe rigidity as those at risk; in such cases, short-acting benzodiazepines may be drugs of choice. The elderly may also be at risk. A thorough drug history can reveal the patient's attitude and experiences with pharmacologic agents used previously and thus serve as a guideline for future prescriptions.

REFERENCES

1. Anthony, E. J. Childhood depressions. In Depression and Human Existence, E. J. Anthony and T. Benedek (Eds.). Little, Brown, and Co., Boston, 1975.

2. Ayd, F. J., Jr. (Ed.) Chronic renal lesions: A Hazard of long-term lithium treatment. International Drug Therapy Newsletter, 12:37—40, 1977.

3. Beck, A. T. The Diagnosis and Management of Depression, Univ. Pennsylvania Press, Philadelphia, 1978.

4. Cole, J. Antidepressant drug treatment. In Clinical Handbook of Psychopharmacology, A. DiMascio and R. I. Shader (Eds.). Jason Aranson, New York, 1970.

5. Feighner, J. P., Alden, G. C., Fabre, L. F., et al. Comparison of alprazolam, imipramine, and placebo in the treatment of depression. J.A.M.A., 249:3057-3064, 1983

6. Glassman, A. H., Kantor, S. J., and Shostak, M. Depression, delusions, and drug response, Am. J. Psychiatry, 132:716-719, 1975

7. Gram, L. F., and Fredricson-Overo, K. Drug interaction: Inhibitory effect of neuroleptics on metabolism of tricyclic antidepressants in man. Br. Med. J., I:463-465, 1972.

8. Greenblatt, D. J., Allen, M. D., and Shader, R. I. Toxicity of high dose flurazepam in the elderly. Clin. Pharmacol. Ther., 21:355-361, 1977.

9. Greenblatt, D. J., Shader, R. I., and Abernethy, D. R. Drug Therapy: Current Status of Benzodiazepines (Part 2), New England J. Med., 309:410-416, 1983.

10. Gross, H. S. Depressive and sadomasochistic personalities. In Personality Disorders, J. R. Lion (Ed.). William & Wilkins, Baltimore, 1974.

11. Gulevich, G. D. Convulsive and coma therapies and psychosurgery. In Psychopharmacology: From Theory to Practice, J. D. Barchas, P. A. Berger, R. D. Ciaranello, and G. R. Elliott (Eds.). Oxford University Press, New York, 1977.

12. Hollister, L. E. Clinical Use of Psychotherapeutic Drugs. Charles C. Thomas, Springfield, Ill., 1973.

13. Hollister, L. E., Motzenbecker, F. P., and Degan, R. O. Withdrawal reactions from chlordiazepoxide (Librium). Psychopharmacologia, 2:63-68, 1961.

14. Hollister, L. E., Overall, J. E., Pokorny, A. D., and Shelton, J. Acetophenazine and diazepam in anxious depressions. Arch. Gen. Psychiatry, 24:273-378, 1971.

15. Jefferson, J., and Greist, J. H. A Primer on Lithium. Williams & Wilkins, Baltimore, 1977.

16. Kales, A., Allen, C., Scharf, M. B., and Kales, J. D. Hypnotic drugs and their effectiveness: All-night EEG studies of insomniac subjects. Arch. Gen. Psychiatry, 23:226-232, 1970.

17. Kales, A., and Kales, J. D. Recent advances in the diagnosis and treatment of sleep disorders. In The Relevance of Sleep Research to Clinical Practice, G. Usdin (Ed.). Brunner/Mazel, New York, 1972.

18. Klein, D. F., and Fink, W. Psychiatric reaction patterns to imipramine, Am. J. Psychiatry, 119:432-438, 1972.
19. Klerman, G. L. Modes of action of antidepressant drugs. In Pharmacotherapy of Depression, J. O. Cole and J. R. Wittenborn (Eds.). Charles C. Thomas, Springfield, Ill., 1966.
20. Kotin, J., Post, R. M., and Goodwin, F. K. Drug treatment of depressed patients referred for hospitalization. Am. J. Psychiatry, 130:1139-1141, 1973.
21. Lennard, H. L., Epstein, L. J., Bernstein, A., and Ransom, D. C. Hazards implicit in prescribing psychoactive drugs. Science, 169:438-441, 1970.
22. Lesse, S. Psychotherapy in combination with antidepressant drugs in the treatment of patients with marked depressions. In Masked Depression, S. Lesse (Ed.). Jason Aranson, New York, 1977.
23. Lion, J. R., Azcarate, C., and Koepke, H. Paradoxical rage reaction during psychotropic medication. Dis. Nerv. Syst., 36:557-558, 1975.
24. Morris, J. B., and Beck, A. T. The efficacy of antidepressant drugs. In Progress in Psychiatric Drug Treatment, Vol. 2, D. Klein and R. Gittleman-Klein (Eds.). Brunner/Mazel, New York, 1976.
25. Ostow, M. Psychological considerations in the chemotherapy of depression. In Depression and Human Existence, E. J. Anthony and T. Benedek (Eds.). Little, Brown, and Co., Boston, 1975.
26. Post, R. M., Carbamazepine's acute and prophylactic effects in manic-depressive illness: an update. Internat. Drug Therapy Newsletter, 17:5-10, 1982.
27. Prien, R. F., and Caffey, E. M., Jr. Long term maintenance drug therapy in recurrent affective illness: Current status and issues. Dis. Nerv. Syst., 38:981-992, 1977.
28. Rickels, K. Drug treatment of anxiety. In Psychopharmacology in the Practice of Medicine, M. E. Jarvik (Ed.). Appleton- Century-Crofts, New York, 1977.
29. Risch, S. C., Janowsky, D. S., and Huey, L. Y. Plasma levels of tricyclic antidepressants and clinical efficacy. In Antidepressants: Neurochemical, Behavioral, and Clinical Perspectives, S. J. Malick and E. Richelson (Eds.), Raven Press, New York, 1981.
30. Schou, M. Preparations, dosage and control. In Lithium: Its Role in Psychiatric Research and Teatment. S. Gershon and B. Shopsin (Eds.). Plenum Press, New York, 1973.
31. Shader, R. I., Greenblatt, D. J., Salzman, C., Kochansky, G. E., and Hartmatz, J. S. Benzodiazepines: Safety and toxicity. Dis. Nerv. Syst., 36 (Suppl.):23-26, 1975.

CHAPTER 3

Behavior Disorders

The behavior disorders are among the largest group of conditions seen in clinical practice. They present the therapist with many challenges in treatment due to their destructive nature and the fact that the therapist so often feels helpless about activity he cannot control. Behavior disorders range from impulsivity among children to antisocial acts among adults. These behaviors appear quite heterogeneous; at first glance, it would seem that childhood hyperkinesis is quite different from adult criminal activity. However, target symptoms often have a common denominator and include low frustration tolerance, lability of mood, and aggressiveness. With the exception of minimal brain dysfunction, studies concerning pharmacologic treatment of these symptoms and behaviors is largely uncontrolled in nature. Since there is no one drug specific for these conditions, it is necessary for the clinician to conceptualize the etiology of the behavioral syndrome and treat the underlying state. This state may be that of minimal brain dysfunction, an epileptoid condition, an affective disorder, or hypersexuality. These diverse clinical entities will be discussed separately.

Alcoholism and drug addiction are ubiquitous disorders of mankind and form a large bulk of practice also. In both disease processes, there is orientation toward the procurement of a drug, its excessive use, and the development of dependency. Target symptoms have a common denominator which include drug hunger. Varying modalities of therapy have been seen as useful for the abortion of such hungers but have met with limited success for no drug agent fully quenches these drive states.

Finally, patients may be brought to clinical attention who suffer from specific tics, phobias, or problems with enuresis or nightmares.

These are generally a disparate group of entities. Pharmacologic control is idiosyncratic and not based upon a target symptom concept. Rather, drugs useful for these disorders have been found by serendipity; the disorders will be mentioned briefly as specialized problems for intervention.

An 8-year-old boy was referred for evaluation because of psychomotor restlessness at school, low frustration tolerance with temper outbursts, and poor learning. He had difficulties with his attention span and demonstrated mirror image writing. There was a history of some birth trauma but minimal delay in developmental milestones. The remainder of the history was unremarkable.

On mental status examination, the patient appeared as a restless and distractable young boy who would not sit still during the interview and fidgeted and paced around the room, randomly picking up toys and discarding them. Subsequent neurologic evaluation revealed some evidence of reflex asymmetries and difficulties with coordination.

A diagnosis of hyperkinesis secondary to minimal brain dysfunction was made. The patient responded to dextroamphetamine (Dexedrine) 10 mg b.i.d. and was kept on this regimen for 9 months. The medication was discontinued at the end of the school year.

The above case is a fairly typical example of such cases seen in pediatric and child psychiatry settings. Children who demonstrate poor school performance as well as disruptive behavior disorders often arrive with a diagnosis of minimal brain dysfunction already made by a non-medical observer. Within recent years, there has been increased sensitization on the part of the public to this diagnosis. Such sensitization has led to two types of reactions. The first involves an overdiagnosis of the syndrome with requests for medication by those who must live with and teach the child. The second involves a concern on the part of parent or civil rights groups regarding the excessive use of medication to treat these children. The opposing groups view medication as abhorrent and see little role or justification for drugs in childhood. As with most things, a reasonable position is one between both extremes.

The diagnosis of minimal brain dysfunction is a difficult one to make. Hyperkinesis, a term used to refer to the psychomotor component of the syndrome, is rather nonspecific; the majority of cases of hyperkinesis seen in clinical practice are probably functional in origin and reflect emotional difficulties. For these cases, drugs are not indicated. When, however, the hyperkinesis is associated with signs of organicity as detected on psychological testing and neurologic examination, then a diagnosis of minimal brain dysfunction may be somewhat more easily made.

Yet there are other problems in the evaluation. Many children are restless the first time they see the doctor. Several visits to the clinician may be indicated. The setting is also important. Some children are calm at home and restless in school or *vice versa*. Thus, the clinician asked to see a child in a structured environment may find him quite tractable, only to be told by agonized parents and teachers alike that he is unmanageable elsewhere. In some cases, a visit to the school by the clinician is advantageous. Third party observation weighs heavily in the diagnosis and must be sifted by the clinician. Some children recognize that they are overly restless and easily distractible and thus view their hyperkinesis as dystonic. This may help with the diagnosis.

Yet hyperkinesis is not always evident in cases of minimal brain dysfunction. Some children demonstrate only distractibility and poor attention span in the classroom setting without marked psychomotor activation. Recognition of this is seen in DSM III formulations where the diagnosis "Attention Deficit Disorder" can be used with and without the term "Hyperkinesis."

The assessment of cortical dysfunction is problematic. The psychologist must be sensitive to tests of fine visual-motor function and impulsivity. The neurologist, likewise, must be interested in cortical dysfunction and the subtle apraxias and coordination difficulties these children show. If consultants simply administer standard psychological tests for IQ determination or evaluate a child for signs of gross focal neurologic findings, the subtle signs of minimal brain dysfunction may be missed. Distractibility, low frustration tolerance, impulsivity, and aggressiveness are parameters of psychomotor activation and form an important set of target symptoms suitable for pharmacologic control (10). Many of these symptoms are available on checklists which can be given to parents and teachers to ascertain the efficacy of therapy. Actually, teachers are often the most dispassionate and fairest observers of progress because they are less biased and prejudiced than parents, have less guilt about the child's difficulties, and have a much larger sample of children as a comparison group for any one child's behavior.

In various controlled studies, it has generally been found that central nervous system stimulants are more effective than placebo when used on various groups of school children referred because of academic and behavioral problems due to minimal brain dysfunction. These studies have measured improvement by a variety of visual-motor performance tests as well as subjective assessment of target symptoms such as those described above.

As with all drugs in psychiatry, the mechanisms of action of central nervous system stimulants is unknown. One hypothesis is that these medications act on a dysfunctional reticular activating system to make the child more responsive to stimuli which he would otherwise not properly sort out and attend to. In children with minimal brain dysfunction, stimulants produce a quiescent effect and act as normalizers. This is in contrast to normal adolescents and adults, where stimulants lead to behavioral activation. In the latter group, stimulant use leads to tolerance; abuse can result in euphoria, and toxicities, including those of a paranoid psychosis, have been described. In children with minimal brain dysfunction, stimulant use is not accompanied by tolerance and abuse effects are not observed.

The pacification induced by stimulants has been called "paradoxical." Yet it must be remembered that stimulant drugs may also normalize the mood and behavior of depressed children. Thus, the specific response is not diagnostic of minimal brain dysfunction.

The central nervous system stimulants on the market differ principally in terms of potency and duration of action. Methylphenidate (Ritalin) appears to be associated less with growth suppression while dextroamphetamine causes less difficulties with tachycardia; the two are comparable in efficacy (18). Pemoline (Cylert) is a weaker stimulant but has a long span of action and can be given in a single daily dose. There is no way to predict whether or not these drugs will be useful and efficacy of treatment is an empirical matter.

While central nervous system stimulants have been the drugs of choice in cases of minimal brain dysfunction, other drugs have also been used. Generally, the role of antidepressants, antianxiety agents, and antipsychotic medications in the treatment of this syndrome are equivocal and studies have not clearly defined these drugs as effective as the central nervous system stimulants. They may be useful in cases refractory to the latter. Since lethargy is the most frequent side-effect of these medications encountered in children, decrements in cognitive function may result.

In the treatment of minimal brain dysfunction, central nervous system stimulants require titration to clinically adequate dose ranges. These ranges are generally well within those established by the manufacturer. Titration should be carried out assiduously since a small increase may make a large difference in children. Lack of proper titration resulting in undermedication is one of the more common reasons why these drugs are abandoned and labeled as ineffective.

In the above case, the patient initially received 5 mg of dextroamphetamine in the morning. This dose had some ameliorating effects on his hyperactivity. The dose was given after breakfast to delay absorption and to reduce anorectic effects. The patient began, however, to show some hyperactivity after lunch since the drug has an effect of 3 or 4 hours. He thus required a supplemental dose in the midafternoon. Regimens of twice a day are usual; occasionally, a t.i.d. regimen is required. If so, the third dose should be given long before bedtime. Two main problems associated with central nervous system stimulants are their tendency to produce insomnia and anorexia. If patients are troubled by loss of sleep, a b.i.d. regimen can be divided so that two-thirds is given in the morning and one-third in the late afternoon. Insomnia usually remits with time. If it is a continued problem, the antihistamine diphenhydramine (Benadryl) may induce drowsiness safely.

Reduced food intake secondary to the anorectic effects of stimulants may lead to a growth lag, particularly if these drugs are used for long periods of time. Thus, use of stimulants requires that the clinician maintain a height and weight chart in order to ascertain normality of development.

Central nervous system stimulants should be discontinued for short periods approximately every 6 months while the child is in school in order to ascertain continued need. Vacations and summertime are also logical times to withdraw medications in order to counteract growth disturbances and observe behavior. However, vacations may often be more stressful for the child than school, and each case must be individualized. Abstinence is not a simple matter. Teachers are usually very sensitive to the child's medication compliance and can tell easily if he missed the morning dose. The same is also true of other children in the class who often make fun of the child who "forgot his pill."

Those in a position of observing the child at school should be told ahead of time so that they do not become alarmed. Both teachers and parents must also be counselled to be patient as the first several days of abstinence may be the worst, reflective of some behavioral "rebound" which eventually evens out.

The fact that teachers and school officials need to be informed of medication shifts emphasizes the close alliance necessary between the clinician and teachers. Some schools are quite tolerant of minimal brain dysfunction problems; others are not and the therapist may have to spend some time with personnel in some educative efforts.

The rationale of employing central nervous system stimulants is to provide adjunctive pharmacologic control until some degree of physiologic maturation occurs, precluding the need for these drugs. Thus, abatement of target symptoms when the patient is off medication signals the end of medication needs. However, if a child has done well during the summer without drugs, consideration should be given to reinstitution of stimulants when school begins again in the fall. There is a chance that the child may show hyperactive behavior again under this stress and thus skew the teachers' perception of him as being a poorer student than he actually is. Once so perceived, the situation is difficult to change. It is better if the child is able to show maximum potential from the outset. Later, the drugs can be discontinued on a trial basis.

In a schoolroom situation, there is a placebo value in giving drugs to a child who misbehaves or who has difficulty learning. Those around him see that he is getting medication to help him with his temper and learning problems. Often a positive feedback is established and teachers become more receptive to the child, offering him more attention which in turn alleviates the child's condition.

The parents of hyperactive children are often distraught and anxious. This feeling may stem from the fact that they must live with a child who may be a social embarrassment to them. Other anxieties may stem from guilt relating to erroneously perceived child rearing or some defect in parenting. Some of these anxieties are allayed by the statement on the part of the clinician that there exists some degree of brain dysfunction which can be alleviated by a pill. However, additional alarm may arise if the word "brain damage" is utilized to describe these children. Even if the word "dysfunction" is used, it can be heard incorrectly.

The clinician may explain to parents that there appears to be some temporary nervous system developmental difficulty which is biochemical or neurophysiologic in nature and responsible for the child's behavior; in most cases, with treatment, the condition remits in time. However, there is a hazard in placing too much emphasis on biochemistry, for psychological parameters are important and parents may blame all difficulties on the organicity, thus circumventing the need for psychotherapeutic measures. Medication should be described as a small part of the treatment plan. Vastly more important is education with regard to limit setting and the need to make parents think twice about taking their child to places where he may be overstimulated, such as a circus or amusement park. Individual tutoring may be considered for patients with severe learning disabilities. Parents must be sensitized to stop escalating fights among siblings and intervene sooner than they might otherwise, since the child's trigger mechanism is such that anger becomes an all-or-none matter. Parents must also learn how to praise the child for things done correctly; children with minimal brain dysfunction are subject to burdens of medication and correction and need their share of positive reinforcement.

One concern parents have about drugs pertains to the future of drug abuse. Since the medications being given the child are those with abuse potential in normal adolescents and adults, parents may worry that the child will become addicted to the same substances in later life. There is no evidence that this is the case, and discussion about this is reassuring.

With regard to the child's posture of taking medication, it should be remembered that many children have fantasies about physical harm. The attitude with which mothers or fathers give medication is important and may reinforce earlier patterns of being forced to eat or being put in a subservient or subordinate position. There is trust inherent in the process of taking medication and some children can be given the dignity of being allowed to take at least the morning dose of medication. If the afternoon dose is taken in a public place, attention must be directed toward possible ridicule by other children. Some school systems are understanding in this matter and have flexibility so that a teacher can be made responsible for the dose while in other settings the nurse is responsible and available only during specific hours. Each instance may vary and confront the clinician with different strategies of drug administration.

The length of time required to treat minimal brain dysfunction with central nervous system stimulants has not been fully determined. In some instances, the use of these agents continues up to midadolescence, but there is a general feeling among clinicians that the drug should be discontinued by late adolescence and that the disorder should hopefully remit by that time. Yet even if the hyperactivity disappears, there may be sequellae such as learning disabilities and personality disturbances with aggression and poor impulse control. Hence, continued long-term monitoring of the patient is in order, and the clinician must not assume that a simple reduction in those target symptoms which characterize minimal brain dysfunction means the end of the matter.

There have been anecdotal reports of "hyperactive adults" who respond to central nervous stimulants (3). Certainly, one is prone to see adults who do demonstrate the clinical characteristics of children with minimal brain dysfunction. These individuals show the same mood lability, impulsivity, and problems with aggression as their childhood counterparts and are often diagnosed as explosive personalities. Currently, this personality disorder appears in DSM III formulations as one of a class of "Disorders of Impulse Control" and most closely conforms to the entity of "Intermittent Explosive Disorder." This disorder is described as one in which the individual shows sudden and paroxysmal outbursts of rage with rapidly mounting tension and the rapid release of anger. These outbursts are generally out of proportion to the psychological stresses and are accompanied by some alien feelings of guilt or remorse. They are often associated with premonitory changes in sensorium, hypersensitivity to light and sound, and other aura-like phenomenon. The outbursts themselves have a seizure-like quality to them and are accompanied by some degree of amnesia. There may be associated "soft" neurologic findings together with evidence of some organicity on psychological testing and positive electroencephalographic findings.

Because of the "epileptoid" quality to this type of aggression in adults, anticonvulsants have been used in treatment (14). Literature regarding the use of anticonvulsants is not rigorous and generally is anecdotal in nature. However, these drugs may be considered in certain clinical instances where temper outbursts and repetitive rage outbursts do appear to have a strong seizure flavor to them, particularly if they are of relatively recent onset rather than representing the ingrained life-style of the patient (12).

Many psychiatrists are reluctant to use anticonvulsants and have limited familiarity with them. Anticonvulsants are seen as drugs more in the purview of neurologists; there is some reluctance to use them unless there is clear-cut electroencephalographic evidence such as that associated with classic forms of epilepsy. However, it should be recalled that opinion varies widely in this area. Neurologists may use anticonvulsants in the absence of electroencephalographic data which support seizures felt to be present on clinical grounds. Sleep electroencephalographic studies are desirable to induce cortical hypersynchrony and activate limbic system abnormalities thought to be responsible for a behavior disorder. Such findings as 14 and 6 per second changes, although controversial, may provide the indication for anticonvulsant medication.

Other positive findings such as those derived from careful psychological testing may also substantiate organicity and allow the clinican to infer seizure-like brain dysfunction. With regard to neurologic examination, the clinician must take into account that some neurologists are more interested than others in the neurologic aspects of psychiatric disease and in the assessment of cortical dysfunction. The same need to look for "soft signs" for the diagnosis of minimal brain dysfunction is desirable in the adult who demonstrates a paroxysmal behavior disorder. In rare instances, psychomotor epilepsy resulting from temporal lobe dysfunction can be diagnosed; this condition will be discussed later.

Anticonvulsants are generally prescribed for long periods of time. The fact that they must be taken regularly lest withdrawal seizures occur makes patient selection important. To some extent, this is paradoxical since it is precisely those patients with mood lability and impulsivity whom one wishes to treat with a medication they must take regularly. As mentioned previously, this is also the case with lithium. However, anticonvulsants are less toxic than lithium and overdose rarely leads to potentially lethal complications. Furthermore, after a reasonable length of chronic dosing, nighttime consolidation is possible.

The anticonvulsant drug most used in psychiatry is diphenylhydantoin (Dilantin). Diphenylhydantoin has been used in a vast array of psychiatric disorders including thought and affective disturbances; its most rational potential usefulness is in disorders of aggression which have "ictal" characteristics (12). The medication can be given in divided dosages up to the usual amount of 300 to 400 mg per day. After 10 days, adequate blood levels are reached and nocturnal consolidation is possible. As with lithium, phenytoin levels are important in the monitoring phase of treatment and indicate to the physician both compliance and efficacy of the drug. There are patients who metabolize the drug too readily and will require larger than usual amounts. Conversely, some patients do not respond to therapeutic blood levels and must be tried on alternate anticonvulsant regimens. The following case example illustrates this point.

> A 30-year-old woman was referred for evaluation because of temper outbursts directed at her children. The patient related a disintegrating marriage and much turmoil surrounding the issue of anger at her husband. She was prone to disciplining the children overzealously, and occasionally struck them.
>
> On closer scrutiny, the temper outbursts appeared paroxysmal and were accompanied by some minor changes in sensorium before the outburst and subsequent remorse and mild amnesia for the event. There was a history of repeated head trauma in childhood and "hyperactivity."
>
> An electroencephalogram showed occasional 6 per second unilateral spikes. Further neurologic evaluation was unremarkable. A trial of diphenylhydantoin was attempted. The dose was begun at 300 mg t.i.d. and consolidated after 2 weeks in an h.s. regimen. On this level, she achieved a blood level slightly below therapeutic range. Accordingly, the dose was stabilized at 400 mg h.s. There was a fairly prompt reduction in her aggressive outbursts. Further psychotherapy ensued and she remained in treatment for a year during which time she went through a mild depressive episode in the course of the separation and final divorce proceedings.

This case illustrates several aspects of treatment of patients with paroxysmal hostile outbursts. In the above case, the patient had significant problems with impulse control. Her neurologic history revealed possible head trauma and an electroencephalogram revealed equivocal evidence of brain dysfunction. Rigorous documentation of an epileptic process presumed to be etiologically responsible for her temper was lacking. However, it appeared to the clinician that she did indeed have some ictal-like features to her temper and that there were some changes in consciousness which resembled an aura, and amnesia reminiscent of a post-ictal confusional state. On empirical grounds alone, an anticonvulsant was begun.

Had this patient not responded to diphenylhydantoin in therapeutic dose ranges with adequate blood levels, the clinician might have used primidone (Mysoline) as a second choice. The latter drug is somewhat more toxic and associated with a higher incidence of blood dyscrasias.

Carbamazepine (Tegretol) has already been described as a drug useful for the therapy of manic-depressive illness but its utility extends to the treatment of episodic behavior disorders as well, including those characterized by paroxysmal aggressive outbursts thought to reflect temporal lobe pathology (21). Its principal toxicity is bone marrow suppression.

Much has been written about the role of psychomotor epilepsy in psychiatric disorders. Most work indicates aggression to rarely be the manifestation of the actual seizure state but rather a phenomenon seen during the post-ictal confusional period or during the inter-ictal period when there is heightened irritability (5). Yet other observers have described aggressive outbursts which apparently correlate with electro-encephalographic changes seen in patients including those with surgically implanted brain electrodes and are thus persuaded that seizures may manifest themselves in violence (1). The polemic over this matter is somewhat academic for the clinician confronted with the violent patient. In either case, the rationale of using anticonvulsants lies in the reduction of the ictal episode which secondarily reduces the post-ictal period and lessens or abolishes the inter-ictal buildup of tension.

It is often assumed erroneously that temper outbursts must be motiveless and undirected for them to be perceived as ictal and hence identified as treatable with anticonvulsants. Yet the issue lies not so much in the apparent irrationality of the aggressive act as it does in its overdetermined nature and the fact that the act is out of proportion to the psychosocial stress. Even more important is the lability or paroxysmal quality to the aggression which is the most important parameter or target symptoms for pharmacologic control. In the above case of the woman with temper outbursts, it was evident that her anger had a real basis. She was furious with her children on whom she relied upon for affection in lieu of her husband. The children unfortunately were subjected to a "Sunday father" who took them out once a week and spoiled them with gifts and trips. This made the mother very angry and she displaced her anger on the children. It was not so much the content of the anger nor the fact that her anger occurred when the children returned from a visit at the father's home but the suddenness and intensity of the anger which was noteworthy.

The above patient was a reliable historian. Not all patients are and it is difficult to assess the efficacy of drugs used to treat adult patients with temper problems. Unlike thought and affective disorders which persist over time and can be viewed for days, weeks, or months, aggression is a symptom which is often reported by a third party and is phenomenologically one which is viewed only momentarily. With children, observers are present during most of the day. This is not the case with older patients. The hospitalization of these patients often leads to a prompt reduction in their base rates of behavior so that pharmacologic control can not truly be ascertained. When the clinician does use drugs on an outpatient basis he must rely upon some system of keeping track of the frequency of outbursts, their duration, and intensity. Corroboration by another member of the family is often desirable. This can only be done if the clinician recruits a spouse or relative. The issue may compromise confidentiality, but trust is often an issue anyway since the patients themselves often do not report temper outbursts accurately, for several reasons. First, temper outbursts are often syntonic. And second, many of these patients are quite manipulative. If they are in legal difficulties, they may wish to "look good."

The use of drugs in the above case was adjunctive since there was much therapy to be done. The anticonvulsants were particularly useful in aborting the impulsive behavior which led to so much guilt and remorse in the patient. Once the impulsivity was reduced, the patient could effectively deal with the other more substantive issues confronting her which included the loss of her husband and feelings of inadequacy as a mother. Subsequently, a depression ensued which was clinically significant but did not require antidepressants.

Psychotherapeutic efforts must also be aimed at educating the patient into the sequelae of his actions. Attempts must be made to teach the patient to recognize these somatic manifestations of affective states. When angry, the patient must come to identify that anger by becoming aware of the clenched fist, the rapid breathing, the tightness of the stomach, the racing pulse, and other physiologic parameters to which he has not paid attention. Many patients prone to behavioral outbursts have an impoverished ability to recognize their own inner emotions and cannot meditate upon them. Suddenly, the dysphoric state overwhelms them, leading to arguments, drinking, impulsive drug taking, or other actions designed to quench the unpleasant affect. In addition, patients showing behavioral problems often nave an inability to fantasize (15). This leads to rapid and impulsive behavior without foresight as to the consequences. Therapeutic efforts must be directed toward creating within the patient an increased ability to foresee the outcome of behavior. Some patients who act impulsively literally act before they think; that is, the motor component of behavior dominates their life. Generally, they have handled anger in an outwardly direct fashion. With pharmacotherapy, such pathways are less available to them. Hence the anger is often internalized and patients complain of being overwhelmed by more "feelings" than they have ever been in their lives. This is but the first step in the long verbal psychotherapeutic process (11). To some extent, it should be predicted to patients that drugs will hopefully stop their outbursts but at the same time will lead them to experience more emotions and even sadness which they used to handle by striking out. As is seen in pediatric psychiatry, it is often "easier to be mad than sad" and the same concept identified in children is applicable to adults who suffer from temper tantrum problems. To a large extent, the depression resulting from the diminution in aggressive outbursts is reminiscent of the postpsychotic depression mentioned previously. Thus, the abandonment of projective defenses in behavioral styles leaves the patient to mourn such processes and come to grips with a good deal of inner reflection which is initially dystonic. It requires a certain amount of ego strength to adhere to this psychotherapeutic regimen and treatment is obviously not suitable for severely disturbed character disorders who are so labile as to never be able to settle into any introspective process. Postures of depression are often equated with weakness. In some cases, this principle is amenable to therapy while in other cases it is not and the patient flees from further self-discovery and abandons treatment.

Another problem which may occur is similar to the phenomenon seen in children whose behavior difficulties are perceived as being organic and hence not directly under their control. Thus, for some adult patients, administration of a drug to control temper takes the matter "out of their hands," so to speak, and exonerates them from efforts to control deviant actions.

The excessive use of aggression generally betrays weakness and vulnerability and the clinician must recognize this. Individuals prone to rage and excessive hostility are often vulnerable and fragile people whose self-esteem is tenuous and quickly shattered. Brittle reaction formations against underlying helplessness give way when any kind of significant verbal challenge ensues. This psychodynamic formulation should alert the clinician to the problem of self-esteem which is often the core psychological difficulty in these patients. As poor self-esteem surfaces in therapy, it can be mistaken for depression and antidepressants may be prescribed. It is better, instead, to alert the patient to the fact that it will take time to work through bad feelings about the self and that there is really no specific medication for this venture. If despair becomes intolerable and the patient is at risk for leaving therapy, small amounts of antianxiety drugs may convey an attitude of caring.

Just as depression can occur when aggression is blocked, so, too, can worsening personality changes and irritability develop with increased seizure control. Instead of a psychodynamic explanation, some workers have conceptualized this inverse relationship to reflect seizure control which is still imperfect but only appears to be in remission (13). For example, patients who are still tense and irritable will not be able to relax during electroencephalographic evaluations. This, in turn, may lead to a spuriously normal electroencephalogram since sleep does not occur; as mentioned, a sleep-activated electroencephalogram is an optimal way of eliciting temporal lobe dysfunction. The clinician viewing the unremarkable electroencephalogram may conclude that the seizure state is improved but the patient's irritability has worsened. In reality, dose adjustments may be necessary. Still other clinicians feel that the curtailment of seizure states does lead in some manner to a damming up of emotions and recommend periodic withdrawal of anticonvulsants to allow a controlled seizure to occur (5).

This situation remains unresolved and is mainly theoretical. It would appear to be most logical to use anticonvulsants during the early stages of treatment until some insight is obtained and the patient acquires the skill to deal psychologically with affect and anger. Then, the drugs can be withdrawn on a trial basis. Reinstitution may be necessary in some instances although it must be recalled that chronic use of anticonvulsants may lead to other toxicities such as cerebellar changes (16). Thus the patient must be monitored.

Some of the above-mentioned verbal psychotherapeutic strategies are luxuries for the extremely provocative adolescents seen in practice. Here, defiance precludes psychopharmacologic treatment and the case is usually that the patient is already experimenting with his own street drugs. While there are abundant target symptoms of irritability, impulsivity, and aggressiveness, a therapeutic nihilism prevails. The clinician with an orientation and known repute for using medications in practice may be at a disadvantage; when intense countertransference feelings of anger and helplessness make the physician reach too quickly for drugs in an attempt to quench the belligerence he sees, he should consider referring the patient to a colleague whom the adolescent recognizes as more likely to engage in dialogue. This tactic may reduce struggle for power and dominance and allows a therapeutic alliance to develop.

The term "acting out," is often used to describe patients prone to unmanageable behavior. Strictly speaking, the term is a transference related one referring to the fact that the emotions generated between patient and therapist, unconscious or unarticulated, become translated by the patient into behavior outside of the therapy. In general parlance, "acting out" is used for any form of undesirable behavior. Yet the clinician should recall that strong emotions evoked in treatment may well propel the patient toward self-destructive, aggressive, or sexual behaviors which are seemingly random but may well reflect the relationship the patient has with the former therapist.

It would be an oversimplification to think that anticonvulsants are the only drugs for aggression and impulsivity. In previous chapters, the use of antipsychotic and antianxiety agents has been mentioned as useful for their respective underlying thought and affective disorders which may give rise to aggression. In addition, lithium carbonate has shown some utility in the treatment of aggression and isolated literature has shown it to be better than placebo in the treatment of certain prisoners prone to hostile outbursts (20). The reason for the utility of lithium here is unclear. Certainly, lithium has no direct antiaggressive effect though its antimanic properties may be useful to calm certain excited patients who are hypomanic and manic. More likely, the explanation for the efficacy of lithium lies in the fact that it is being used to treat an atypical affective disease state manifested not by the usual cyclical swings of depression or elation but by changes in levels of irritability and psychomotor activation. Thus, aggressive patients responding to lithium may be those with an undiagnosed manic-depressive illness who during the "high" phase show an increased tendency to become belligerent, hostile, and irritable. During the "low" phase, the same patients then show psychomotor retardation with some apathy and indifference. As mentioned previously, lithium is a poor drug to give to labile and impulsive individuals. Hence, its use is generally confined to those individuals who are hospitalized or incarcerated or otherwise in situations where drug use can be monitored.

Sexual aggressiveness may be brought to the attention of the clinician. The aggressiveness in this instance is a special form associated with sexual arousal. The heightened drive state seen in patients prone to such behaviors as pedophilia or repeated rape has been treated with thioridazine with the rationale of capitalizing on the propensity of this drug to produce impaired ejaculation as a side-effect. This tactic is questionable from the psychodynamic standpoint since patients who are concerned about their masculinity are apt to be more upset, not less, as they take an agent which still allows sexual arousal but interferes with its orgiastic culmination. A secondary rationale of antipsychotic drug utilization is the interference with libido which accompanies long-term use. This effect is idiosyncratic and hence questionable, since long-term antipsychotic drug use for non-psychotic conditions may produce other toxicities. A more potentially rational pharmacologic approach to the problem of hypersexual aggressiveness involves the use of hormonal blocking agents or female hormones. When administered in depot form to men, there results a significant lowering of serum testosterone with a secondary reduction in sexual arousal and fantasies. While there exists a literature in this work, control studies are lacking and these drugs are still considered experimental (4). The matter is mentioned to alert the therapist to the fact that the target behaviors of sexual aggressiveness are currently difficult to treat with existing psychopharmacologic agents. Currently, behavioral deconditioning and more conventional psychotherapeutic approaches are the most that can be offered to patients. Adjunctive antianxiety medications may be useful occasionally for more motivated patients who become excited and translate that excitation into sexual arousal which leads to adverse sexual behavior.

As problematic for pharmacologic treatment as sexual deviancy is alcoholism. To some extent, the two behaviors are common in that a heightened drive state leads to an abnormal behavior. In the case of sexual deviancy, the individual is repeatedly propelled to engage in some destructive behavior. There are compulsive mechanisms driving him to engage in ritual, and the fulfillment is incomplete and intermittent, leading to repetition. Alcoholism has similar properties. Alcoholics are prone to drink and repeat their drinking patterns in an attempt to obtain some form of gratification. The analogy between the conditions of sexual deviancy and alcoholism may help the clinician understand psychopharmacologic approaches used in both illnesses. Basically, attempts have been made to interfere with the drive state with the hope that patients will thus be no longer prone to behave adversely.

Like all addictive behaviors, alcoholism bespeaks an underlying conflict which drives the individual to drink. The conflict may be visible, covert, or hypothesized. In some instances underlying anxieties or agitations or depressions are perceived as target symptoms amenable to pharmacologic control. This accounts for the wide use of antianxiety, antipsychotic, and antidepressant agents in the treatment of alcoholism. These agents are used with the rationale that they will produce a substitutive or restorative state, thereby freeing the alcoholic from the need to use the beverage for sedation or tranquilization. Unfortunately, this paradigm rarely works. The same drugs such as the benzodiazepines which are used for cross-tolerance during the acute withdrawal from alcoholism have severe limitations for maintenance phases of the same illness. The orality of the alcoholic has been described and, like the borderline patient, there exists a need to fill a psychological emptiness. This need is profound and constitutes a hazard in psychopharmacologic management. Alcoholics are prone to use drugs together with their alcohol for increased disinhibitory effect. Thus, the drug is taken conjointly with alcohol, rather than instead of it. Alcohol is a unique pharmacologic agent which induces pleasurable disinhibitory sensations together with a euphoria. No drug can easily match this. In addition, there are powerful social and psychological parameters which are associated with drinking so that it is not just the alcohol itself which is desired but the social stimuli as well. People drink in bars to meet others and the taste cures and social expectations powerfully shape behavior.

Various agents which interfere with the metabolism of alcohol have been used to produce aversive effects in those predisposed to drink. Such a strategy is designed to lead to a deconditioning and extinguishing of drinking behavior. Disulfiram (Antabuse) interferes with the metabolism of alcohol. One of the metabolic breakdown products, acetaldehyde, produces a wide range of highly unpleasant symptoms including tachycardia, nausea and vomiting, and dizziness, and has an associated morbidity and mortality. Therefore, the drug cannot be used in patients who are chronically ill or have cardiovascular or hepatic difficulties. Furthermore, the tablet must be taken daily. Because this is the case, the alcoholic can simply not take the medication and relapse. Those who do adhere to a regimen of disulfiram are obviously a select group of alcoholics motivated to stop drinking.

Despite these nihilistic comments, there is still need on the part of the clinician to ascertain the underlying condition of the alcoholic since alcoholism is a symptom as well as a disease process (2). In some instances, evidence of a thought disorder exists and the alcoholic is evidently using alcohol to medicate himself much as a schizophrenic might utilize antipsychotic medication in the context of a clinic setting. In other instances, alcoholism may reflect an underlying depression which is handled by drinking. The following case example illustrates this.

> A 35-year-old housewife with many marital difficulties was prone to daytime drinking and the neglect of her children. After several months of intermittent psychiatric help, she injured herself physically in the house and was hospitalized. In the confines of the hospital, she admitted to a severe despondency and showed the hallmarks of a depression with psychomotor retardation, apathy, tearfulness, and insomnia. An antidepressant was begun and maintained subsequent to her release from the hospital with a cessation of her drinking behavior.

This example illustrates the potential of detecting the underlying and affective disorder which leads the patient to drink. Unfortunately, the clinician must recognize that alcoholism is more than self-medication as indicated above but represents, in addition, a more malignant psychopathologic process having to do with chronic problems with self-esteem and identity. Thus, intensive psychotherapeutic work is necessary to avoid relapse since the particularly potent effects of alcohol do prove a temptation for patients who have disturbances with intimacy and object relations and are prone to drink as a means of filling an inner emptiness. The powerful peer group pressure exerted by self-help groups such as Alcoholics Anonymous are often distinctly advantageous for these patients who require a strong supportive milieu and ritual to bind anxieties.

It should be noted in the above case that abstinence was necessary before the clinician could make the diagnosis of depression. While patients are drinking and only intermittently sober, they rarely admit to their true states and careful evaluation of the premorbid personality and the additional history furnished by relatives or friends may be vital. Hospitalization may prove ultimately to be the best way of seeing the patient in a normative state where baseline functioning can be assessed.

It may be extremely difficult to remove alcohol from a patient and deprive that patient of something so ubiquitously available. The underlying depression and despair which has motivated the patient to drink initially must be dealt with through some form of psychotherapy. Again, no one drug suffices in this venture.

The problem of drug hunger exists with narcotics addiction. Strategies of using cross-tolerant drugs form the bases for the treatment of addiction much as is attempted for alcoholism (22). Methadone maintenance programs depend upon the supervised use of this synthetically produced narcotic to protect the patient against the illegal use of street narcotics he may otherwise use to get "high." Methadone by itself induces a feeling of comparative comfort without euphoria when stabilized maintenance levels are attained. In theory, the idea of methadone maintenance is good, although generally these measures have met with limited success. Superimposed illegal narcotics, particularly when given intravenously, can still induce a euphoria. Thus, no narcotic substitute program makes the patient immune from a "high" which can be induced by the addition of another agent, including additional quantities of methadone. Obviously, the illegal narcotic would have to be extremely potent and of very pure properties to produce such a high given the significant dose used in methadone maintenance programs and it is unlikely that any street dealer would carry such high quality substances. Patients do "chip" and use alcohol, the barbiturates, or other hypnotics or sedatives including the benzodiazepines to induce some transient altered state of consciousness; cross-tolerance does not exist with these drugs.

Methadone maintenance is not simple and confronts the clinician with administrative policies to which he must adhere. For example, FDA guidelines require documentation of addiction of at least 2 years duration; this can be ascertained clinically in the basis of needle tracks and abscesses and/or a history of treatment in community hospitals. In addition, the patient must have had a documented attempt at detoxification. Finally, the patient must show some signs of withdrawal. If these qualifications are met, the patient who comes in "off the street" with a history of drug use is eligible for methadone as a substitute. Methadone is titrated upward to a maintenance level of 50 to 100 mg per day. There is a range of opinion regarding the optimum upper limit. Lower dose limits give the patient less to sell on the street, a temptation for patients who take home a weekend's supply when the clinic is closed. Higher limits may be dictated by the patient's procurement of other drugs, an indication that drug hunger is not yet satisfied. To a large degree, the clinician depends on outside behavior to determine when the optimum blockade dose of methadone is reached. Methadone has a relatively short half-life and requires daily administration in liquid form. Newer drugs with longer half-lives are currently under investigation. Longer acting compounds would preclude the daily attendance on the part of addicts at clinics although some workers feel that clinic attendance and the social rehabilitative programs of clinics are as much the treatment process as the drug itself. As is the case with alcoholism, there are a powerful set of social reenforcers operative in narcotic addition. The use of a needle, a street culture, and other parameters associated with peer group pressure and the procurement of drugs powerfully influence the behavior of addiction. No pharmacologic agent is specific for these many psychological variables and methadone, while curbing the target symptom of a "drug hunger" or the "appetite" of the user, must be supplemented by intensive therapy programs.

An alternate experimental pharmacologic strategy is to use a narcotic antagonist such as naltrexone which induces blockade of illegally administered opiates so that they have no effect. The difficulties with these drugs are that they do not alleviate drug hunger and are thus not taken reliably by patients unless the latter are extremely well motivated. In this respect, use of these agents is similar to the use of disulfiram in alcoholism and requires a good deal of motivation. Disulfiram, of course, produces an aversive reaction while narcotic antagonists simply make the use of heroin a neutral venture.

In an earlier paragraph regarding the use of central nervous system stimulants to treat hyperactive children, mention was made of ethical questions raised about the utilization of this drug on populations of children. A different kind of ethical concern is raised when the clinician uses one narcotic to treat a patient who uses another narcotic. In a sense, the clinician is utilizing a controlled addictive program with the rationale that he is improving the quality of life of an individual who otherwise might illegally look for money to obtain drugs which are impure and are taken in unhygienic fashion. These concerns are unlikely to be resolved. What is known, however, is that the clinical outcome of the patient on methadone maintenance is imperfect. The next case illustrates deeper underlying problems in patients treated with methadone.

> A 28-year-old man enrolled in a methadone maintenance program was seen in consultation because of problems with aggression. He revealed a past history of poor impulse control and temper outbursts in childhood and young adult life. He had killed another man and has been acquitted on the basis of legal insanity. He was a paranoid man, prone to rage when esteem was threatened. Street drugs controlled his temper to varying degrees.

The above patient showed severe problems with hostility which in part accounted for his use of narcotics, drugs being observed to have some pacifying effect. However, the curtailment of addiction was only the beginning of therapy for this man, who subsequently entered intensive individual psychotherapy. Deep underlying character pathology emerged; the addiction was but a symptom of his difficulties (23).

Aggression is one symptom observed among patients in methadone maintenance clinics; another is hunger, already described for the alcoholic. In early stages of treatment and attendance, patients make many demands on the clinicians and seem insatiable in their needs for nurturance. This makes the therapist become quite "giving," a posture which in time has a wearing effect.

Another phenomenon seen in methadone patients also comes as a function of time. Methadone patients frequently show apathy, boredom, and lethargy, symptoms reminiscent of the depression seen in psychotic patients who are ill for years. It is not uncommon to see patients initially enthusiastic over methadone treatment but who, after several years, become "burned out" much as chronic schizophrenic patients do. The etiology of this effect remains undetermined and whether the observation reflects a drug effect or is a matter of psychopathology is unknown. A countertransference problem may develop as staff become dismayed and angry at the lack of enthusiasm of the therapy of young persons who would seem to have a higher potential than they actually demonstrate. Provisions must be made for staff to engage in additional professional activities which negate therapeutic nihilism and are conducive to morale.

An additional burden is placed on the physician and staff by virtue of the policies of methadone maintenance clinics. Here, urine tests are taken to determine whether or not the patient is using illicit drugs such as amphetamines, barbiturates, narcotics, and quinine, the substance used to dilute street heroin. The laboratory approach to the problem of dishonesty is accompanied by a chronic skepticism about the patient's life style as the clinician must constantly be on the lookout for needle marks, constricted pupils, and other aspects of addiction. These factors also shape a more hostile attitude which makes the clinician doubt volunteered data. In psychiatry, the clinician has a certain gullibility and depends upon the introspective material and fantasy life of a patient as the material upon which the therapy is based. With addicts, suspicion is the rule and manipulation supervenes above therapeutic efforts, at least in early stages of therapy until a relationship develops.

The therapist's posture with regard to addictive patients varies considerably from patients having affective or thought disorders. In the latter two groups, compliance may be a problem but generally there exists a reasonable therapeutic alliance. With alcoholic patients and drug addicts, the physician may often find himself functioning as a policeman; such a posture is reinforced by the fact that the alcoholic is always suspect of imbibing and the addict suspect of using illegal drugs. Such vigilance may revert to a form of cynicism and a certain toughness and hardening on the part of the clinician. The latter then assumes a demeanor reflecting the need to avoid being tricked or fooled. This outlook has a direct effect on the use of psychopharmacologic agents. Those clinicians used to working with addictive personalities may be quite sparing and even withholding in their use of antianxiety or antidepressant drugs since the patients they see do not have true despondencies but are always manipulating in order to get drugs.

One solution to this problem is to diversify caseloads so that the clinician sees more classically neurotic patients or even takes some addictive personalities into intensive psychotherapy so as to develop a better appreciation for the inner lives of such patients. In this way, the therapist can keep his professional image and be gentler with patients than he might otherwise be.

There remains for discussion several disorders seen in childhood. These are mentioned because of the fact that specific pharmacologic agents are indicated in treatment and often induce remission. In this respect, they differ from the addictive disorders mentioned previously for which no drugs are specifically curative. The childhood behavior disorders to be described do, however, resemble the addiction in that they may be associated with psychopathology which must also be treated.

Enuresis may be brought to the attention of the clinician. Controversy exists over many aspects of this entity, including age parameters and the significance of primary versus secondary wetting. The latter occurs when a child wets after he has attained the ability to be dry. Psychopathology has been seen traditionally as etiologically implicated for enuresis, although some workers view the phenomenon as a neurophysiologic maturational disorder, since it generally remits with time or medication (6). Psychotherapy may be useful to deal with guilt in children or parents; in some instances when the enuresis is clearly of a reactive nature due, say, to the birth of a sibling, therapy may also be helpful. Most cases, however, do not show clear-cut psychodynamics and are best treated with medication. The drug of choice is imipramine. Other antidepressants may work, but this tricyclic remains the most tested and effective agent. The drug is usually given in a single dose before bedtime.

The mechanism of action of imipramine remains unclear (8). Anticholinergic effects do not appear to be responsible for improvement as anticholinergic drugs more potent than imipramine have not been as effective in the treatment of enuresis. Control studies exist, thus ruling out placebo effects. One possibility is the antidepressant effect of imipramine. Yet, imipramine usually takes several weeks to work in adults while enuresis often responds within the first day or first several days of treatment. More recent work has shown imipramine steady-state plasma levels to occur more rapidly in children and appear within a few days. Other controlled work isolating the antidepressant factor has shown the latter to play a role in therapy. The appropriate way of conceptualizing enuresis remains unclear; what is clear is the frequent empirical response of the condition to imipramine.

Regimens of imipramine should be time limited and abstinence periods should be attempted. Several months of therapy are the rule and improvement should occur within a relatively short time without the need for vigorous titration beyond recommended dosages. If enuresis recurs, another trial can be attempted. If the patient is still unresponsive, alternate treatments such as behavior conditioning paradigms are indicated.

School phobia is another condition causing much anguish in a family. Here, the child suddenly refuses to attend school and demonstrates anxiety and panic at the prospect of going to school, leaving home, or leaving his parent. This form of separation anxiety has been viewed as a psychiatric emergency and traditional treatment methods have focused on prompt and forced return since the longer the child stays away, the more reinforcing the avoidance behavior becomes. Within recent years, a pharmacologic approach to this problem has been attempted. This approach is based upon the utility of imipramine and the experimental treatment of adult agaraphobics who are conceptualized as having some form of separation anxiety responsive to the antidepressant. In control studies, school phobic children have also been responsive to imipramine and have returned to school (7).

The manner in which the drug acts is unknown. At first glance, it would appear that school phobia might be another depressive equivalent. Certainly, children appear despondent and ashamed. Moreover, the separation anxiety can prevade other aspects of their lives and affect socialization with other children. Thus, the child becomes embarrassed and seclusive. He may also become insomniac in anticipation of the next day. Precipitants for school phobias are often losses or changes in the environment.

However, workers utilizing antidepressants for both adult panic states and childhood phobic conditions stress that both populations of patients are not classically depressed as they do not have vegetative signs of depression. While the description of children in the above paragraph would appear to contradict such contentions, the answer may be that childhood manifestations of depression are quite different from those seen in the adult situation and that even in adults, atypical depressions may exist which are pharmacologically responsive. Thus, the panic state of both the adult and child phobic may resemble separation anxiety and may be a circumscribed depressive episode with strong agitated flavoring reminiscent of panic and fear of loss of control seen in certain severely depressed patients. This matter is bound to remain unsettled; the issue is for the clinician to capitalize upon what empirical knowledge there is about the specificity of drug response and consider that pharmacologic agent. Imipramine for the treatment of school phobia should be regarded as experimental. High dosages, including those in the adult range, have been reported as necessary. Thus, the use of the drug would require extreme vigilance if undertaken.

Insomnia has already been mentioned in a previous chapter. There remains the group of dysomnias which can be problematic for the clinician. These include sleepwalking, night terrors, and narcolepsy. Sleepwalking and night terrors are seen primarily in children. These conditions are not apt to be associated with underlying psychological conflict and represent true disorders of arousal from the deep stages of non-rapid eye movement (NREM) sleep, referred to as stages three and four. Somnambulists must be protected from injury and hazardous obstacles should be removed from the room and the child should be protected from falling. Night terrors must be distinguished from nightmares. Nightmares are common in all ages and occur during REM sleep when dreaming occurs most frequently. Recall occurs, and the patient can awaken. Night terrors are reflected in trance-like states of fright without awakening; the child returns rapidly to sleep and has no recall for the event.

While sleepwalking and night terrors appear to be maturational disorders which remit with time, medication may be indicated. In theory, drugs of choice are those observed in electroencephalographic studies to suppress stage four NREM sleep. These are the benzodiazepines, such as diazepam (9). Regrettably, the effectiveness of these agents is inconclusive.

A similar situation exists for narcolepsy, a specific hypersomnia. Here a certain class of drugs, the central nervous system stimulants, may be effective, but the efficacy of agents such as methylphenidate is compromised by the inevitable development of tolerance which comes from long-term treatment. Thus, the clinician may withdraw the drug and begin the patient anew at a lowered dose or try an alternate stimulant (24). As is the case for minimal brain dysfunction, drugs are adjunctive and occupational adjustment is necessary. Exposure to machinery must be minimized.

It must be recalled that most hypersomnias are psychogenic; one of the common causes of excessive sleeping is depression.

A final behavior which shows drug response specificity is the tic referred to as Gilles de la Tourette Syndrome, a condition manifested by involuntary muscular movements which can be associated with verbal utterances such as coprolalia (19). Onset occurs usually during childhood or adolescence. The drug of choice is haloperidol; the drug is titrated to effective levels and lower maintenance regimens are used for as long as the disorder persists. Years of treatment have been described, raising the possibility of long-term toxicity from the drug itself. The effectiveness of haloperidol for this rare condition remains unexplained but is presumed to be a fortuitous interference with deranged brain neurotransmitters. Newer high potency drugs may offer equal effectiveness without the risk of long-term adverse reactions but have not been studied.

Other neurologic movements such as chorea or athetosis may in part resemble Gilles de la Tourette Syndrome, and it is tempting to look at other tic-like behaviors of childhood and adult life as possibly responsive to haloperidol. For example, in one study, some aspects of stuttering improved with use of the drug (17). However, while tics are common, most are treated with much difficulty and do not respond to any medication. Furthermore, it must be remenbered that many disorders of voluntary movement are exacerbated by drugs capable of inducing neurologic reactions. Tics are usually representative of underlying emotional conflict and warrant psychotherapy. Antianxiety agents may play some adjunctive role in certain instances.

REFERENCES

1. Bach-Y-Rita, G., Lion, J. R., Climent, C. E., and Ervin, F. R. Episodic dyscontrol: A study of 130 violent patients. Am. J. Psychiatry, 127:1473–1478, 1971.
2. Beebe, J. E., III. Evaluation and treatment of the drinking patient. In Psychiatric Treatment: Crisis, Clinic, Consultation, C. P. Rosenbaum, and J. E. Beebe, III (Eds.). McGraw-Hill, New York, 1975.

3. Bellak, L. Psychiatric states in adults with minimal brain dysfunction. Psychiatr. Ann., 7:575–589, 1977.
4. Blumer, D., and Migeon, C. Hormone and hormonal agents in the treatment of aggression. J. Nerv. Ment. Dis., 160:127–137, 1975.
5. Blumer, D. Temporal lobe epilepsy and its psychiatric significance. In Psychiatric Aspects of Neurological Disease, D. F. Benson and D. Blumer (Eds.). Grune and Stratton, New York, 1975.
6. Cohen, M. W. Enuresis. Symposium on Behavioral Pediatrics, Pediatr. Clin. North Am., 22:545–560, 1975.
7. Gittleman-Klein, R. Pharmacotherapy and management of pathological separation anxiety. In Recent Advances in Child Psychopharmacology, R. Gittleman-Klein (Ed.). Human Sciences Press, New York, 1975.
8. Greenberg, L. M., and Stephans, J. H. Use of drugs in special syndromes: Enuresis, tics, school refusal, and anorexia nervosa. In Psychopharmacology in Childhood and Adolescence, J. M. Weiner (Ed.). Basic Books, New York, 1977.
9. Kales, A. and Kales, J. D. Sleep disorders: Recent findings in the diagnosis and treatment of disturbed sleep. N. Engl. J. Med., 290:487–499, 1973.
10. Katz, S., Kishore, S., Gittleman-Klein, R., and Klein, D. Clinical pharmacological management of hyperkinetic children. Int. J. Ment. Health, 4:157–181, 1975.
11. Lion, J. R. The role of depression in the treatment of aggressive personality disorders. Am. J. Psychiatry, 129:347–349, 1972.
12. Lion, J. R. Conceptual issues in the use of drugs for the treatment of aggression in man. J. Nerv. Ment. Dis., 160:76–82, 1975.
13. Monroe, R. R. Episodic Behavioral Disorders. Harvard University Press, Cambridge, Mass., 1970.
14. Monroe, R. Anticonvulsants in the treatment of aggression. J. Ner. Ment. Dis., 160:119–126, 1975.
15. Nemiah, J. C., and Sifneos, P. E. Affect and fantasy in psychosomatic disorders. In Modern Trends in Psychosomatic Medicine, O. W. Hill, (Ed.). Butterworths, London, 1970.
16. Reynolds, E. H. Chronic antiepileptic toxicity: A review. Epilepsia, 16:319–353, 1975.
17. Rosenberger, P. B., Wheelden, J. A., and Kalothkin, M. The effect of haloperidol on stuttering. Am. J. Psychiatry, 133:331–334, 1976.
18. Safer, D. J., and Allen, R. P. Side-effects from long-term use of stimulants in children. In Recent Advances in Child Psychopharmacology, R. Gittleman-Klein (Ed.). Human Sciences Press, New York, 1975.
19. Shapiro, A. K., Shapiro, E., Wayne, H. L., Clarkin, J., and Bruun, R. D. Tourette's Syndrome: Summary of data on 34 patients. Psychosom. Med., 35:419–435, 1973.
20. Sheard, M. H. Lithium in the treatment of aggression. J. Nerv. Ment. Dis., 160:108–118, 1975.
21. Tunks, E. R., and Dermer, S. W. Carbamazepine in the dyscontrol syndrome associated with limbic system dyscontrol. J. Nerv. Ment. Dis. 164:56-63, 1977.
22. Wikler, A. Treatment of opioid addiction. In Psychopharmacology in the Practice of Medicine, M. E. Jervik (Ed.). Appleton-Century Crofts, New York, 1977.
23. Wumser, L. Mr. Pecksniff's horse: Psychodynamics of compulsive drug use. National Institute for Drug Research Monograph, 12:36-72, 1977.
24. Zarcone, V. Narcolepsy, N. Engl. J. Med. 288:1156-1166, 1973.

CHAPTER 4

Questions and Comments about Drugs

In the previous chapters, attention was directed toward pharmacologic principles and psychotherapeutic strategies of drug use. Also, psychodynamic aspects of pharmacology and illness were discussed. What now follows are some typical questions and comments made by patients who ask for medications, describe side-effects, or wonder about long-term outcomes. The clinician should understand both the manifest and latent content of the material.

"Is there any medication which will help my condition?"

The patient may ask this at the inception of treatment and during the initial interview, or after some time has elapsed in psychotherapy. When mentioned at the outset, the question may be aimed at identifying whether the physician is the type to use drugs. If mentioned during therapy, the question reflects a wish for relief of symptoms but also may signify the patient's desire for a pharmacologic solution to more chronic and deeply ingrained psychological difficulties which give rise to affective disturbances. Sometimes, the questions means: "Am I bad enough to warrant one of those strong drugs I have heard about?" Generally, the clinician should reflect the question back to the patient and ask the latter's views on the matter. A statement by the therapist to the effect that the question is a worthy one acknowledges the patient's sincerity. Thus: "I think your question is reasonable, but I wonder what you feel medications will do for you?" The patient can be asked what he has heard about medications and what specific symptoms he thinks medication will help. Patients may have heard from relatives that certain "magic" drugs such as lithium may make them immune from ever being ill. The patient may also have unrealistic expectations about antidepressant or antianxiety drugs. In some cases, the patient has already experimented on his own with medication or been previously prescribed ineffective doses; the question then is one based upon a certain hopelessness that may have resulted from former experience with drugs. Patients with a history of extensive drug exposure are as apt to ask this question as are pharmacologically naive patients.

The term "any" can be significant when seen during the despair of depression when the patient wishes relief. In reality, the question may mean: "Am I hopeless?"

'Do I have to take this medication?"

Here, the clinician has presumably broached the subject of medication and the patient is showing some resistance. A statement should be made to the effect that the patient appears to have some reservations about the drugs: "You seem to have some concerns about the medication. Can you tell me what they are?" This should elicit underlying fears about side-effects and toxicities, and shame and guilt about the need for medication to begin with. For some patients, medication means that they have succumbed to a severe mental illness. Assurance about drug safety and the relative ubiquity of drug use for emotional difficulties should help in this process.

For some patients, the question about *having* to take the medication has to do with a power struggle. One statement of use is: "No, you don't have to do anything and you are the person who plays the key role in our treatment. Tell me your thoughts about medication." This sometimes brings to light underlying anger at authority figures or the therapist.

"I'm not taking any medication."

This is usually a defiant remark most often provocatively made by patients resisting treatment; rarely, it may be uttered by a patient already in therapy who becomes defensive upon the introduction of the idea of using drugs. The issue is one of control. The patient is saying: "No one will control my mind by outside forces through the use of drugs."

It is presumed that the therapist has either thought through the reasons for suggesting medications and strongly favors drugs or is simply hearing the patient's remarks for the first time. In the latter instance, a useful comment is: "You obviously don't have to do anything you don't want to, including just coming to see me. The choice is yours and you're the boss. However I'd be curious about your reasons for the decision." This comment acknowledges that it actually is the patient who is in charge, a fact that the latter often appreciates; defusion of the power struggle may result from such discussion.

For patients in treatment, the sudden emergence of this statement signifies alarm at the introduction of a variable the patient feels he cannot control. The patient may see discussion as safe and even comfortable, but the adjunctive use of drugs escalates the matter beyond what he is used to. In other words, the statement is: "I can deal with our talking together, but medication may make you master of me." The clinician must address himself to whatever trust is available to the relationship since the alliance is usually fragile and threatened by the issue of medication. A statement such as: "You seem to have strong feelings about drugs. Yet we've been talking together and gotten along pretty well. Do you feel that medication will do something to change that?" In some instances, the introduction of medication turns out to signify to the patient that his dignity has suffered and that he will be just another one of "those zombies I see in the hospital." The fantasies are complex and warrant exploration.

It is difficult to convince recalcitrant patients to take drugs, and the clinician may often feel that it is almost not worth it. Sometimes it pays to say this directly: "Look, you are a difficult patient and have your own ideas on medication. I think this drug will help you, but I can't force you to take it. If it alienates us, it isn't worth fighting over." Within this sentence is a statement of how the drug might help the patient; this must be detailed. If the drug is used for a behavior disorder to control impulsivity, the rationale of use should be spelled out. For antipsychotic drugs, clarification of the effects of the drug on thought processes requires careful and open discussion. "The haloperidol I want to give you will decrease what I observe to be suspiciousness. I know that you don't agree with me all the way on this and we see things differently. That's OK. You can think about trying the medication and watching other people's reactions to you as well as your own level of anxiety. Then see what you think—I'd value your opinion since you have to decide."

Children are often asked to taste a little bit of medication they do not like or want. This regressive maneuver sometimes works with adults as well. Patients can be asked whether they would try a little of the medication to test its effects. If, as previously mentioned in the chapter on antipsychotic drugs, no untoward effect ensues, there may be relief so that the patient can himself titrate the drug to therapeutic levels. Again, it is always desirable to avoid overwhelming a patient with medication.

"What are some side-effects of this medication?"

The physician is always in a quandary when answering this question for too much information may evoke untoward reactions in hysterical patients and inadequate preparation may jeopardize drug therapy with paranoid or obsessional individuals who discard the drug when an unpredicted effect occurs. Generally, the question can in part be reflected back to the patient such as: "I'd be pleased to answer you, but I wonder what specific concerns you have about the medication." Sometimes, this remark targets an area of anxiety such as sedation, addiction, or the like. The clinician is best off being honest but still withholding mention of all effects since no one's interests are served by an exhaustive list of everything that can possibly go wrong with the use of the drug. A reasonable position to take is: "Let me tell you some of the common reactions that people sometimes have when they use this medication." The patient can then be told predictable side-effects such as dry mouth or blurred vision. At the same time, he must be told that such effects are expected properties of the drug, and do not mean that the medication is causing a "reaction" or an "allergy;" patients have many confusions about side-effects as opposed to toxicities.

For patients at risk, more specific information is desirable. "It may happen that you get dizzy when you use the medication. This doesn't mean that something is going wrong—give me a call and tell me about it so we can adjust the dose." As future sessions with the patient take place, he may have more questions about long-term effects and comes to trust the clinician more in these matters.

"Can't you give him some medication, doctor?"

This comment is often made by relatives on behalf of the patient who may be acutely psychotic or in the early stages of decompensating. Often, the family is agitated and desperately wants help in controlling a malignant process they see unfolding before their eyes. Sometimes, relatives make the request long before the patient himself asks about medication. This may be natural when the illness is syntonic for the patient and dystonic for the family. However, the fact that the family asks first brings up the issue of control; some family members want the patient tranquilized in order that the family equilibrium can be preserved. The question should eventually be reflected on to the patient even thought it can be acknowledged with those who ask. Thus, the clinician can state that there are, indeed, medications available but that he would like to hear the patient's opinion about the same question. Differences of opinion may signal family discord which is apt to play a role in the dispensing of drugs at home. Battles can ensue over the patient's "taking his medication."

Families may also complain that the patient is undermedicated and ask that he be given a higher dose. Again, the dynamics of this request need to be assessed and the clinician must also spend time with the patient alone.

"The medication makes him feel bad."

Again, this statement reflects the subordinate role of the patient and the dominance of a spouse or another family member. Often, family members are the first to comment on toxicities which the patient should be responding to. When this does not happen, the patient, in an individual session, can be asked why he himself did not think about asking of side-effects and toxicities. An underlying theme in this statement is concern about the assertiveness or anger which comes with patient improvement. For many families, improvement of one member may signify a shift in the status quo so that other members become alarmed at the change and register this alarm by making an urgent comment as to side-effects. They may be covertly asking that the medication be stopped.

An alterate explanation should always be considered; namely, that the toxicity is subtle. Akathisia is an example.

"My husband doesn't like the pills I'm taking."

This comment has many underlying meanings. The husband may be very angry at the patient's illness, not the fact that medication is required. Additionally, the husband may begrudge the individual psychotherapy sessions and wish that the patient would confide in him, rather than in a therapist. This comment is one, then, of jealousy regarding the intimate relationship between the therapist and patient. In general, patients making this comment need to be asked how the spouse feels about the patient's illness and what exactly the husband is saying about the medication. Usually, medication is not so much the issue as the illness. In some cases, spouses have certain concerns about long-term effects of medication or have read about such matters. If this is the case, a conjoint session may be useful in putting to rest certain fantasies or fears about these drugs.

An alternate hypothesis is much more covert. The patient herself may be complaining to the husband about psychotherapy, pill taking, or some attitudes of the therapist, but cannot relate these sentiments to the latter. She thus acts them out so that the husband becomes angry; the message from him is correct but incomplete. She is in effect saying "I do not like the therapy."

"The pills you gave me make my mouth dry."

Since medications produce many side-effects and toxicities, such a statement may in part be real but often has to do with the perception that it was the pills "you gave me" and not just any other kind of medication which produced an adverse effect. As such, the patient is disappointed or angry with the physician and there may exist some unrealistic expectations of drugs or therapy which can be profitably discussed in treatment.

For some paranoid patients, the statement may reflect deeper fears about poisoning although such concerns are usually not amenable to insight unless the therapy is intensive and the alliance strong.

"The medication isn't working."

This remark may reflect impatience if made early in the course of pharmacologic therapy. Or, it may be a manifestation of irrational wishes attendant to the therapeutic process. Patients often seek a feeling of satiation or satisfaction from the therapist much as they may have yearned for nurturance when they were ill at former times in their lives. Unfulfilled longings may surface as transference statements. The patient is saying: "You are not giving me what I need."

When appropriate as dictated by the course and intensity of treatment, the patient can be asked what his expectations of the therapy actually are. Thus: "You are telling me that the drugs I prescribed aren't having a desired effect. I wonder if there is any other aspect of therapy which you find dissatisfying besides the medication?"

"How long will I have to stay on this medication?"

This is a complex query which has been touched upon in the previous text. Patients may have many mixed feelings about reductions in medication or abstinence from medication. Concern about withdrawal of the physician's attention, or the discontinuation of treatment may be the issue. Alternately, the patient may be wishing for more verbal interaction with the therapist. Thus, the question is really: "Can you spend more time with me instead of giving me pills?"

Another possible underlying concern is the availability of the therapist. Thus, the question may really translate into: "How long will you be around to take care of me?"

Many patients do wish to know about long-term effects and toxicities but are embarrassed or frightened to ask for fear of hearing something unpleasant. The question reflects denial, in part; in reality, the concern is: "If I stay on these pills a long time, what can happen to my body?" The question is best addressed by acknowledging the patient's seriousness: "That is reasonable to question and I am not sure exactly how long medication will be necessary. But I wonder whether you have some concerns about using any medication for a long time?" Hopefully, this should open the door for dialogue.

Sometimes, the question really is a request: "Please don't take me off the pills because I may get sick again." Attention to this latent interpretation is important. Fear of decompensation is common but not verbalized because the patient is afraid that the doctor will view drug dependence as dangerous and intensify efforts to wean the patient from medication. What the patient is really seeking is reassurance that he must and may stay on the drug longer. Allied to this type of concern is some ambivalence about getting well and relinquishing a sick role. Thus, the patient is afraid of recovery; the question really is: "When it comes time to stop the medication, will I be able to face the real world?"

"Will I become addicted to the medication?"

This is a very common question. Since patient cannot distinguish between antianxiety, antidepressant, or antipsychotic drugs, there is a natural tendency to worry about reliance, dependency, and addiction. Generally, the principle extends to all drugs used in psychiatry since the patient feels that any medication which affects the mind may lead to some kind of pathologic dependency. The truth and fallacies to this should be discussed. More often, the patient is concerned about relying on a medication and preoccupied with how much he will have to use it and for how long. Concerns about the control and passivity may be dormant issues. The question is also asked by individuals who are frightened of medication and fearful that they will lose control or somehow be subjugated by not only the drug but also its usage. Finally, the patient is possibly equating addictive potential with chronicity of illness. Thus, the question really is: "Will my illness last so long that I will never be able to be without drugs?"

"Can I take other medication with this pill?"

Again, this is a more global question relating to drug int. action. Antihypertensive medication, diuretics, hypnotics, and anticonvulsants are types of medications that do not combine well with those used in psychiatry and each case must be individualized. Actually, the physician should have inquired beforehand what medications the patient is taking in order to give the patient proper instruction about drug use. When a patient asks this in a more global manner and is currently on no medication other than what he is receiving or about to receive from the clinician, the query bespeaks underlying concerns about the potency of the drug being given him. Thus the question really is: "Will this drug be so strong that I can never take anything else for any other condition?" Patients often have also some latent embarrassment about having to tell their internist or gynecologist about the fact that they are receiving an antidepressant or antipsychotic drug; this can be discussed with the patient in time also.

"How fast will the pills work?"

This is a rather typical question asked by a patient at the onset of treatment. On one level, the question is a genuine one asking for symptomatic relief. On another level, the patient is asking about the power of medication and the therapist's aid in alleviating a dysphoric state. Some patients may be exceedingly impatient and want immediate drug action. Hence, they will be disappointed easily and it behooves the clinician to spend some time in finding out how fast the patient thinks the medication ought to work. For other patients afraid of being overwhelmed and rendered lethargic too quickly, the question is one of concern regarding the onset of action of the drug.

"Can I drink when I am on this medication?"

This is but one of many questions patients have about drug interaction. A large number of patients enjoy some form of alcoholic beverage with meals and the question does not connote latent or overt alcoholism. Patients most likely to ask these types of questions are those with obsessive-compulsive character structure who are very fearful of cumulative sedation. Generally, the clinician should inquire as to the level of alcohol use and its role. Beverage alcohol with meals is permissible provided that the patient does not become intoxicated or euphoric or suffer from sedation when medication is superimposed. It might be wise to counsel the patient to take one-half the amount of beverage he usually uses to test the drug interaction.

Sometimes, patients who do not drink ask this question to ascertain how strong the drug is and whether an untoward reaction would result from use of the drug plus alcohol.

"If I skip a dose, can I make it up by taking two of the pills?"

This question is one of pharmacokinetics and also has latent meanings regarding compliance. The patient may be telling the physician that he is prone to miss dosages in which case attention must be directed at the patient's propensity to deviate from proper regimens. Other patients do genuinely forget pills and wonder whether they can tolerate a double dose by taking two instead of one. The clinician must assess whether sedation will be a problem or whether other toxicities such as nausea may result from, say, a double dose of lithium.

Sometimes there is a latent test implicit in the question: The patient is really asking how strong the drug is by determining what a threshold level for toxicity will be. Suicidal patients may often subtly try and find out the lethal level of a drug. Sometimes, questions are more overt such as: "If I accidentally take more than one pill, will it harm me?" The clinician must ascertain whether the patient is indeed flirting with ideas of taking too much medication.

"Should the medication be taken before or after meals?"

This question is more often thought about driving home than in the office. Many obsessional patients or even those who are depressed and need a ritual to adhere to will wonder and agonize over whether they should take the pills before or after eating. Generally, the toxicities of medication are somewhat attentuated by prior food intake which slows absorption. Thus, there is a pharmacologic principle that needs to be discussed with patients. Other patients crave detailed directions regarding drug use and such need reflects their compulsive nature. A comment from the clinician such as: "You seem to have some questions about the proper schedule and use of drugs" may elicit other underlying anxieties. Some patients want strict dietary measures to accompany drug use in the manner of a ritual which will both bind anxiety and enhance, in some magical way, the effectiveness of the drug itself.

"Will I get drowsy from the medication?"

This is one of the most common questions asked in practice and reflects many concerns. Most patients do not wish to be rendered lethargic and do wish to have work capacity preserved. They also want to be able to take part in their family and not appear drugged or "zombie-like." On the other hand, some patients with addictive propensities do wish some altered state of consciousness and the clinician will need to make some judgment in this regard. It is often useful to answer the question directly, and then to ask the question: "I wonder whether other medications have made you feel drowsy and what your reactions have been in those instances?" This question about drug history gives the clinician some index of paradoxical reaction to drugs and lets him know the psychodynamics attendant to drug use or misuse.

"Is the drug new? How long has it been used?"

This question has several facets. First, the patient may wish something "new" and relatively powerful since newness is equated with potency. Some patients have had extensive experience with drug use and are looking for something new on the market although these patients generally know full well what new medications exist and to some extent are testing the clinician. Other patients are frightened of new medications and prefer the older ones they have heard about. Some patients have concerns about being used as "guinea pigs" for newer drugs which the clinician does not have experience with. Thus, the real question is: "What is your experience with the medication you are giving me?"

"Can I drive with this medication?"

If the patient does not ask this question, the physician should determine the patient's use of a car and urge caution. Most drugs in psychiatry have some sedative effect. Hence patients must go slowly and test themselves. It is useful to instruct them to see how drowsy they feel in the morning after breakfast. If they feel alert, they can drive. An exception to this would be if the regimen requires a morning dose of a drug, in which case the patient must first observe himself before making a decision.

Patients may operate machinery at work or for pleasure. The same principles apply.

Hypotensive effects of drugs may play a role; this must be kept in mind, particularly with older patients.

"Is the medication expensive?"

This question may not be asked of the individual practititioner as much as it is in clinic settings; embarrassment may play a role. Although a mundane matter, costs for long-term medication mount and not all patients have insurance which covers medication. Generic prescribing is the best way to lower costs of drugs, but patient confusion not uncommonly results from being given a drug the patient is not familiar with. Most patients know Librium; few are acquainted with chlordiazepoxide and many will become alarmed and feel that they have not been given the correct prescription. This situation will become more confusing in the future as other manufacturers compete to make the same generic product.

Education is the answer to this problem. Patients can be told that many companies make the same drug and call it a different name: "I am going to write down the chemical name of the drug I want to give you. The pharmacist will give you the least expensive brand of that drug." Equipotency and purity are concerns of some patients who want the "genuine" or "original" drug; many of these are obsessional patients who cling to a specific name or brand they trust or have heard about. The main point is that the patient not be surprised when he sees an unfamiliar label on the bottle. To this extent, the generic name can be written down on a piece of paper. Thus, the patient can compare this with the drug container label and see that, indeed, they are the same. Some patients need to be told whether the medication is a pill or a capsule. For example, lithium comes in both forms. Patients used to one form may become alarmed when they receive another.

The above concerns may seem excessive, but they are important for paranoid patients who look for inconsistencies to vindicate their mistrust of the world.

Other psychological parameters may play a role. Patients' views of costs may mirror deeper attitudes about themselves. Thus, some patients may want "expensive" medication while others look for bargains and hunt for the cheapest; esteem may be an issue. Some patients ask for sample and want something from the doctor himself, almost in the manner of a gift.

"I stopped taking the medication you gave me."

This statement is not uncommon and reflects a compliance problem. The patient may be angry at the therapist and say it by not taking the pills that "you gave me." In many cases, the statement reflects anger at being placed in a passive posture of taking medication. Since relatives are telling the patient to "shape up," another demand by the physician to the effect that the patient take the pills may be the last straw and the anger at family members may be displaced onto the clinician.

In some instances, the comment is transference related and refers to the fact that parents used to force the patient to take food or other substances which he did not wish to take. This may be the case for certain borderline individuals or psychotic patients.

In other instances, the patient makes the statement as a matter of defiance. The patient is thus stating that "no matter what you do, I will not comply." The tone of the message is passive-aggressive in nature since the patient evidently did not refuse the medication to begin with but stopped taking it on his own. Generally, the comment is hostile in nature and an appropriate interpretation must be made. However, these are generally underlying issues and do not emerge until therapy is well underway.

Sometimes the patient will confide in the therapist the fact that he has not been taking his medication for several weeks or several months. This is an interesting revelation centering around trust and punishment. To a large extent, the patient wants to see how the therapist will react and how angry he will become. Will the patient be discharged? Will the therapist be humiliated that he has been duped so long? Generally, the appropriate comment is geared toward getting the patient to elaborate on the fantasies surrounding this secret transgression. Thus: "You've evidently had this secret inside you for some time. I wasn't aware of your behavior and can easily be fooled by patients—this seems to have been important to you. Can you tell me why?" Or, a statement about the physician's response is useful, such as: "I wonder how you feel I should react?" The clinician must be truthful in his response, for the patient will detect it anyway. Being truthful does not preclude reflecting back on the patient the latter's behavior and its psychological origin.

"I think I am better. Can I stop my pills?"

Here the patient is asking two things. First, he is asking if he really is well; he is not sure. For the statement is that he "thinks" he is well; he is not sure. Patients are often desirous of the therapist's reaction to their condition and want to be told when they are better. They are used to having the physician make pronouncements about their condition or objective statements about recovery. Yet the matter is quite different in psychotherapy, where it is really the patient who decides in large measure when improvement ensues. Progress is not easily gleaned by the clinician's simple inspection of the patient and time must be spent on deeper inquiry into all levels of functioning and hopes for functioning. This is an educative process for many patients. It can also be a dignified experience for the patient, who has never had the full opportunity to express himself about the subtleties in his mood or thinking. Failure of the patient to take some initiative in this regard and make the physician the judge of all improvement may say something about the patient's self-esteem.

The second thing the patient is asking is whether or not he can stop the medication. There are several parameters to consider here. Some patients want to stop pills as soon as they detect early improvement and do not understand the concept of maintenance dosage or prophylaxis. Others wish to "test" their bodies and see how strong they are and how they can resist illness by stopping all medication. Adolescent and paranoid patients may halt drugs to maintain vigilance.

There may be a deeper meaning to the question about improvement and stopping. The patient may be asking what will happen after he is better and medication is stopped. Thus, the question could be: "What is the future of the therapeutic relationship?" This interpretation and allied concerns were discussed in association with a previous question: "How long will I have to stay on this medication?"

The patient is asking whether he can stop the medication. Obviously he can. Thus, there is an issue of permission implicit in this question. The therapist is endowed with an authoritarian image and this is quite natural in the process of rendering care. However, the issue of asking for permission and the relationship between patient and therapist may be germane here. Thus, the doctor can ask the patient: "You seem to be asking my permission to discontinue medication. Obviously, you must have thought about doing this on your own. I wonder what has stopped you?" Such a comment may open the door for discussion about the transference.

"Will the medication change the color of my urine or stools?"

A rare question but one which attests to the patient's propensity to watch his urine or bowels for signs of change of discoloration. Many patients see drugs as quite potent and possessing the ability to influence body mechanisms. They thus wait for any signs suggestive of such change and see it as either good or bad. Few drugs in psychiatry produced marked changes in the color of urine or stool although most drugs can produce constipation and lithium can produce changes in urinary frequency. Thus, patients may be counselled to the possibilities of these reactions and told how to take corrective measures. Often, the question bespeaks concerns about the enormity of change from the medication. Thus patients are really asking "how powerful will these drugs be and can I see the changes in my body resulting from them?"

There are a number of other questions which are often not asked by patients. For example, patients have concerns as to how, say, antipsychotic drugs will effect sexual performance. They may have heard remarks regarding the side-effects of these compounds but are embarrassed to ask. It is incumbent upon the clinician to consider bringing up this matter by stating something to the effect: "Are there some other perhaps more embarrassing questions you have about the side-effects of these medications?"

Many patients have no questions at all about medications but take them in a perfectly acquiescent manner, passively accepting prescriptions without ever commenting upon them. After the clinician has noted this to be a recurring behavior, he might comment on the fact that the patient appears to have no verbal concerns about the medication, something which is unusual. There are a number of possibilities which must be considered. The first is that the patient compliantly takes all medications much as he accepted other things in his life given him by his parents. There may be underlying resentment or a simple inordinate need to be the subservient member of a dyadic relationship which is part of therapy. Sometimes, patients do not use their medication at all and avoid discussing it by not ever making any comments about prescriptions or pills. Silence is as much a message as hypochrondriasis; the patient who says nothing about medication he receives is giving the message that he does not wish to talk about it or is frightened to discuss the matter.

Some words should be said about the process of prescribing. The clinician who has a prescription pad on his desk shows the patient that he is ready to prescribe. When there is no prescription pad, the patient must take a certain initiative in asking for medication. The lack of a prescription pad often brings up issues regarding M.D./non-M.D. differences since patients, even sophisticated ones, do not understand the difference between psychologists and psychiatrists. In part, this may reflect issues about competence, and the need to see the therapist as someone familiar with medicine and medical illness.

The clinician may chose to write the prescription at the end of therapy or early in the therapeutic hour. The latter allows for some discussion, while the former precludes talking about the transaction. When the prescription is torn off the pad and handed to the patient as both parties rise to terminate a session, little can be said until the next hour. Sometimes, the last 10 minutes of the hour can be devoted exclusively to the issue of medication to allow more probing of the matter.

Clinicians often have many concerns that they appear professional and not use source books or the *Physicians' Desk Reference* in the course of prescribing. Yet even the most seasoned therapist will need to look up toxicities, available dosages, the color of tablets, or drug interactions. Books can be consulted in front of the patient. Often, this is more reassuring than it seems and shows the physician to have some humility and a willingness to learn about matters. It is better for the physician to state honestly that he does not know and look something up than to pretend the opposite, something the patient always senses anyway.

Telephone calls about medication may be problematic. Patients may call up and request refills, asking that the clinician phone them in. If the need is genuine and, say, several days or a week will elapse before the prescription can be rewritten in person, such a request is justified; however, the clinician must ask at the next session why the patient forgot to ask for drugs. Such forgetting may signify a desire to get along without pills or represents denial about illness or the severity of illness. Some patients call up a few days before their appointment; the dynamics in such a case may relate to the patient's need to see if the doctor is available or interested in them. Some patients like to call the physician at home to hear what his wife or children sound like or to somehow gain access to the physician's "other life." This should be kept in mind.

Patients show a need for rapid gratification; as their bottle becomes "empty," they wish it filled. While such an interpretation may represent rather deep and unconscious material, it can occasionally be discussed, particularly if the pattern repeats itself.

Other individuals like to have lots of medication in reserve and even others want plentiful supplies for potential overdosages. The dynamics of each case need to be assessed.

When the physician refuses to refill a prescription, anger may ensue. This may be profitably discussed, although the clinician should have a reason in mind for not complying with the patient's wish and so state his thoughts.

Index

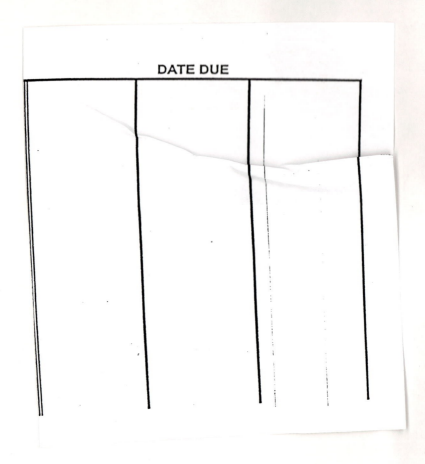

DATE DUE